Smart but Scattered

SMART but SCATTERED

The Revolutionary "Executive Skills" Approach to Helping Kids Reach Their Potential

Peg Dawson, EdD
Richard Guare, PhD

THE GUILFORD PRESS
New York   London

© 2009 The Guilford Press
A Division of Guilford Publications, Inc.
72 Spring Street, New York, NY 10012
www.guilford.com

Printed in the United States of America

This book is printed on acid-free paper.

Last digit is print number: 9   8   7   6   5   4   3   2

Library of Congress Cataloging-in-Publication Data

Dawson, Peg.
    Smart but scattered : the revolutionary "executive skills" approach to
helping kids reach their potential / Peg Dawson, Richard Guare.
        p.   cm.
    Includes bibliographical references and index.
    ISBN 978-1-59385-987-9 (hardcover : alk. paper)
    ISBN 978-1-59385-445-4 (pbk. : alk. paper)
    1. Parenting.   2. Executive ability in children.   3. Children—Life skills
guides.   4. Child development.   5. Parent and child.   I. Guare, Richard.
II. Title.
    HQ755.8.D39 2009
    649'.1526—dc22

                                                          2008026078

Contents

PART III
Putting It All Together

Introduction

There's nothing more frustrating than watching a son or daughter who has so much to offer struggle with the typical tasks and functions of everyday life. The other kids in the class can write down the third-grade homework, remember to take the math book home, and then finish the assignment before bedtime. Why can't your daughter do that? When you sit with her, it's clear she can do the math, and the teacher confirms that she understands the work. Most kindergartners can sit with the class at circle time for 10 minutes without causing major disruptions. How come your son, who's been reading since pre-K, can't stay there for more than 10 seconds? You have an 8-year-old who cleans his room with minimal fuss, but for your 12-year-old the chore sets off a weekly war. Your friends' children don't forget permission slips, lose expensive coats, or fall apart in public. Why does yours?

You know your son or daughter has the brains and the heart to succeed. Yet teachers, your friends, maybe your own parents, and that nagging little voice in your head all say the child isn't where he or she should be. You've tried everything—pleading, yelling, cajoling, bribing, explaining, maybe even threatening or punishing your child to get him to buckle down and do what's expected of him or muster up the self-control to act his age. Nothing has worked.

That's because what your child may lack is *skills*. You can't talk children into using skills they don't have any more than the right incentive could get you safely down a black diamond run when you can't even ski the bunny hill. Your child may very well *want* and have the potential to do what's required but just doesn't know *how*. Scientists who study child development and the brain have discovered that most children who are smart but scattered simply lack certain habits of mind called *executive skills*. These are the fundamental brain-based skills required to *execute* tasks: getting organized, planning, initiating work, staying on task, controlling impulses, regulating emotions, being adaptable and resilient—just about everything a child needs to negotiate the typical demands of childhood in school, at home, and

1

with friends. Some kids lack certain executive skills or lag behind in developing them.

Fortunately, there's a lot you can do to help. This book will show you how you can modify the daily experiences of a child aged 4 to 14 to build the executive skills that will make it possible for the child to get on track and get things done. The groundwork for the development of executive skills in the brain is laid before birth, and you can't control this biological capacity. But neuroscientists now know that these skills develop gradually and in a clear progression through the first two decades of life. This gives you infinite opportunities throughout childhood to boost the executive skills your son or daughter seems to lack.

With the strategies you'll learn in this book, you can help your child learn to clean her room, get homework done, wait her turn, handle disappointment, adapt to unexpected changes in plans, manage new social situations, follow directions, obey rules, save her allowance, and much, much more. You can help your son or daughter meet the thousands of other large and small demands that are part of a child's life and reverse an alarming pattern of falling behind in school, losing friends, and generally falling out of step with peers.

We've seen the methods in this book work for thousands of kids in the school setting and back at home with their families. The strategies require a certain commitment of time and consistency, but none of our methods is difficult to learn or adopt. Some you may even find fun. There's no doubt that these alternatives to constant supervision, nagging, and cajoling will make your *lives* together more fun.

What Can This Book Do for You and Your Smart but Scattered Child?

At some point, to some degree, all children struggle with getting organized, exercising self-control, and getting along with others. Battles over room cleaning erupt regularly in almost every home in the United States. And there isn't a 13-year-old on the planet who does all his homework flawlessly, with perfect promptness, every single day. But some kids seem to need constant supervision and help far beyond the point when their peers are beginning to manage certain tasks on their own. You're probably wondering when you're going to be able to retreat to the sidelines like the other parents: When will you be relieved of issuing constant reminders? When will your child learn to calm himself rather than relying on you to do it? Will a time ever come when you can stop stage-managing every event in your child's life to ensure her success?

These milestones may be a long time coming if you bank on a late-bloomer leap in development. While you're waiting, your child could suffer damage to self-esteem, and you will remain frustrated and worried. So if your child doesn't have the executive skills to meet others' reasonable expectations, it makes sense to take action now to help him catch up. Executive skills have recently been identified as the foundation that all children need to negotiate the demands of childhood, and these brain-based skills become more and more critical as children venture into the world with decreasing parental supervision and guidance. Ultimately, they are essential to successful management of adult life. Acting now to boost your child's executive skills could spare the child a lot of difficulty in years to come.

If your 5-year-old lacks or lags behind the other kids in executive skills, he may not be able to stand to lose a game or keep his hands to himself and could end up with an ever-dwindling selection of playmates. If your 9-year-old can't plan her work and then stick to the plan, she may never finish the longer-term school projects assigned at this age. If your 13-year-old has little impulse control, what's to stop him from leaving his little sister alone to ride his bike with the guys just because you're not there to remind him he agreed to babysit? In adolescence, will your daughter pay attention while driving with a car full of friends? Will your son go to SAT review classes or spend his time instant messaging or playing video games? Will your child have the organization and time management skills to get to a summer job on time and the emotional control to avoid blowing up at an annoying customer or boss? Once grown, will your child leave home or "fail to launch"? In short, will your son or daughter be able to lead a successful independent life?

The chances are far, far greater if you help your child build missing or weak executive skills starting now. This is one of the reasons we focus on kids of preschool to middle school age: If you begin to work on your child's executive skills now, by the time she reaches high school you'll have given her an important foundation for success during that important part of her academic and social life. You'll then find that she is armed with greater self-control, decision-making, and problem-solving skills than you might dream of right now. A lot of what we illustrate for middle schoolers may work for your high school son or daughter anyway, but because high school kids face much different executive-skill-related demands and respond to different parental coaching approaches than littler kids, we won't go into depth here on the older age group.

About This Book

As we have worked with other children—and watched our own children grow up—we've found that all kinds of children may struggle with executive skill weaknesses and that what you can do to help will vary depending on the age and developmental level of the child, as well as on your own strengths and weaknesses and which problems are causing you the most trouble. If you can target the right behavior and choose the right strategy, you can have a positive, significant, and long-lasting impact on your children's ability to develop executive skills. Helping you figure out where your child needs help and the best angles of attack for strengthening those executive skills is the main goal of Part I of this book.

Chapters 1–4 provide an overview of executive skills, how they develop, how they show themselves in common developmental tasks, and how you and the environment can contribute to the development of strong executive skills. Different scientists and clinicians have categorized and labeled executive skills in various ways, but all of us in this field agree that these are the cognitive processes required to (1) plan and direct activities, including getting started and seeing them through, and (2) regulate behavior—to inhibit impulses, make good choices, change tactics when what you're doing now isn't working, and manage emotions and behavior to achieve long-term goals. If you look at the brain as organizing input and organizing output, executive skills help us manage the output functions. That is, they help us take all the data the brain has collected from our sensory organs, muscles, nerve endings, and so forth and choose how to respond.

In Chapter 1 you'll learn more not only about the specific functions of executive skills but also a little about how the brain develops, and, more specifically, how executive skills develop in children, beginning at birth. This understanding should give you an idea of how far-reaching the functions of executive skills are and why weaknesses or deficits can limit a child's daily life in so many ways.

To be able to identify your child's particular executive skill strengths and weaknesses, of course, you have to know when the various skills are expected to develop—just like you did for motor skills like sitting, standing, and walking when your child was a baby and a toddler. Most parents already have an intuitive sense of the developmental trajectory for executive skills. We, and our children's teachers, naturally adjust our expectations to fit each child's growing capacity for independence even though we probably don't consciously label these milestones as the acquisition of various executive skills. Chapter 2 will give you a closer look at this trajectory, listing the common developmental tasks that require the use of executive skills at different childhood stages. We'll also show you how executive skill strengths and weaknesses tend to follow certain patterns in individuals, although it's also true that the skills overall may be better developed in some people than in others. You'll begin to form a picture of your own child's strengths and weaknesses with a set of brief tests. This picture will help you start identifying possible targets for the interventions we offer in Parts II and III.

As we've said, a child's biological capacity for developing executive skills is determined before the child is born, but whether the child reaches her potential for developing those skills depends a lot on her environment. You, as parents, are a huge part of your child's environment. This is not to say that you're to blame if your child has executive skill weaknesses, but knowing where your own executive skill weaknesses and strengths lie can enhance your efforts to build your child's executive skills and also reduce conflict that may have arisen due to certain mixes or matches between you.

Let's say your child is very disorganized and so are you. Not only will it be tough for you to teach your child organizational skills, but battles over disorganization may increase exponentially. Armed with knowledge of this similarity, however, you may be able to establish a camaraderie with your child over the shared need to learn these skills. Working on them together can preserve your child's pride and encourage cooperation.

Or imagine you uncover a mix rather than a match: Just being aware that you are by nature superorganized where your child is disorganized can make you feel more inclined to be patient with your child so you can help him build the skill in which you're so strong. It's not that he's just trying to aggravate you, it's a matter of executive skill differences. Chapter 3 will help you understand where your own executive skill strengths and weaknesses lie and how you can use this knowledge in your efforts to help your child.

The fit between you and your child is not the only one you should be looking at. Goodness of fit between your child and the rest of the environment is also important. As you'll learn once you get into the strategies for building your child's executive skills, the first thing you should always turn to when trying to offset an executive skill deficit is altering the environment. Of course you can't do this forever— and a major goal of this book is to ensure you won't have to—but this is exactly what parents do to varying degrees throughout their kids' childhood and adolescence. We put safety plugs in outlets to keep creeping babies from putting curious fingers into electrical outlets; early play dates always involve parents or caregivers staying with the children; we limit our kids' Internet and iPod time so they get their homework done. In Chapter 4 we'll show you how to look at your child's environment for goodness of fit with his executive skills and what kinds of stage-managing you can do until your child no longer needs such environmental supports.

Once you know where your child's strengths and weaknesses lie and what the fit between you and your child and between your child and the environment looks like, you're ready to start working on building those skills. We believe the reason our interventions are effective is that (1) they are applied in the child's natural setting and (2) you can choose from different angles of attack. These choices allow you to custom-tailor your efforts to suit the child you know so well, and they give you a Plan B to try if Plan A isn't entirely successful.

The first chapter in Part II (Chapter 5) gives you a set of principles to follow whenever you're deciding what the best angle of attack is for a particular problem task or a particular executive skill that your child needs. Three of these form the framework for all the work you're going to do, and each of these is described in one of the chapters that follow (Chapters 6–8): (1) make adjustments in the environment to improve the goodness of fit between the child and the task; (2) teach the child how to do the tasks that require executive skills; or (3) motivate the child to use the executive skills already within his repertoire. As you'll see, we generally recommend that a combination of these three approaches be used to ensure success, and Chapter 9 shows you how to put them all together. Meanwhile, you can decide whether you'd like to adopt some of the scaffolding techniques or use some of the games we suggest in Part II to boost your child's executive skills in a seamless fashion during the course of the day.

You'll also want to target certain problem situations that are causing lots of aggravation for all and/or certain executive skills that are causing your child problems across all the domains of her life. Chapter 10 offers teaching routines aimed at the problems most commonly reported by parents of the children we see in our clinical practice. These routines give you a set of procedures, and in some cases a script, that will help your child learn to manage activities of daily living with less effort and turmoil, whether it's following a bedtime routine, handling changes in plans, or tackling a long-term school project. Many parents find it easiest to begin with these routines because they directly address a task that's a source of conflict every day and because we've supplied all the steps and tools you need. You may find this the best way to get used to executive-skill-building work and the shortest route to observable results. Parents need motivation too, and there's nothing like success to keep you going. These routines tell you how to adapt the routine for your child's age. They also identify the executive skills needed to perform that task, so if you find that the same skills are needed for the tasks causing your child the most trouble, you may decide to read and work on those skills in the corresponding chapters that follow.

Chapters 11 through 21 take up each executive skill individually. We describe the typical developmental progression of the skill and give you a brief rating scale you can use to determine whether your child is on target or lagging with respect to skill development. If you feel your child's skills are generally adequate but could use some tweaking, you can follow the general principles we list for how to do this. If you recognize that problems are more pronounced, however, you can create your own intervention, based on the models we provide for a couple of more intensive interventions, focusing on those problem areas that arise most frequently in our clinical practice. These interventions incorporate elements of all three methods described in Part II.

We're confident that, given all these different choices, you'll find a way to help your child build weak executive skills into stronger ones. But we live in an imperfect world, so Chapter 22 includes troubleshooting suggestions for those times when you run into a brick wall, including questions you should ask yourself about the interventions you have tried, as well as guidance for how and when to seek professional help.

As parents, you can help your child use strong executive skills to get homework done and form good study habits, but you can't follow him into the classroom. Most scattered children encounter problems in school as well as at home. In fact it may very well be your child's first teachers who have made you aware of your child's executive skill weaknesses. Chapter 23 offers suggestions for how to work with teachers and the school to make sure your child gets the necessary help and support in school as well as at home. This includes suggestions for how to avoid adversarial relationships with teachers as well as how to access additional support, such as 504 Plans or special education, if needed.

The skills your child builds with your help should help her negotiate school more successfully, but what happens after middle school? For scattered youngsters, high school and beyond present additional challenges—ones that are often scarier to contemplate than when children are younger and you're focused much more on the upside of growing independence. The last chapter in this book offers guidance for helping your child handle the life stages ahead.

For now, we know it's sometimes scary to look down the road and imagine what will happen when your children reach adulthood. We both know that when our oldest sons were in middle school, we had sleepless nights wondering how they would ever make it through high school, let alone to whatever point lay beyond high school. We've written this book in part to assure you that children *do* grow up and learn to make it on their own. Our kids did it—yours can too. Years of clinical and parenting experience went into the writing of this book. We hope you find it helpful, no matter where you are on your child's journey from childhood to independence.

Part I

WHAT MAKES YOUR CHILD SMART BUT SCATTERED

1

How Did Such a Smart Kid
End Up So Scattered?

Katie is 8 years old. It's Saturday morning, and her mother has sent her to clean her room, with the admonition that she can't go across the street to play with her girlfriend until everything is picked up. Katie reluctantly leaves the living room where her younger brother is engrossed in Saturday morning cartoons and climbs the stairs. She stands in the doorway and surveys the scene: Her Barbie dolls are scattered in one corner, a tangle of dolls and outfits and accessories that look from a distance like a colorful gypsy ragbag. Books are piled every which way in her bookcase, with some spilling out on the floor. Her closet door is open, and she sees that clothes have fallen off hangers and drifted to the floor of her closet, covering several pairs of shoes and some board games and puzzles she hasn't played with recently. Some dirty clothes have been kicked under her bed but are visible in the space between the bedspread and the floor. And there's a pile of clean clothes strewn around the floor by her bureau, left there after a mad search for a favorite sweater she wanted to wear to school yesterday. Katie sighs and goes to the doll corner. She places a couple of dolls on her toy shelf, then picks up a third doll and holds it at arm's length to inspect the outfit she's wearing. She remembers she was getting the doll ready for the prom and decides she doesn't like the dress she chose. She scrabbles around in the pile of miniature clothing to find a dress she likes better. She's just snapping the last fastener on the dress when her mother pops her head in the door. "Katie!" she says, a note of impatience in her voice. "It's been half an hour and you haven't done a thing!" Her mother comes over to the doll corner and together she and Katie pick up dolls and clothes, placing the dolls on toy shelves and the clothes in the plastic bin that serves as a clothes chest. The work goes quickly. Mom stands up to leave. "Now, see what you can do with those books," she says. Katie walks to the bookshelf and begins organizing her books. In the midst of the pile on the floor, she finds the latest in the Boxcar Children series, the one she's in the middle of reading. She opens the book to the bookmarked page and begins reading. "I'll just finish this chapter," she tells herself. When she's finished, she closes the book and looks around the room. "Mom!" she cries out plaintively. "This is way too much work! Can I go play and finish this later? Please?!"

Downstairs, Katie's mother sighs heavily. This happens every time she asks her daughter to get something done: she gets distracted, discouraged, and off track, and the job doesn't get done unless Mom sticks around and walks her through each and every little step—or caves in and does it all herself. How can her daughter be so unfocused and irresponsible? Why can't she put off just a little of what she'd prefer to do until she finishes what she *has* to do? Shouldn't a third grader be expected to take care of *some* things on her own?

Katie has been in the 90th percentile on the Iowa achievement tests since she began taking them. Her teachers report that she's imaginative, a whiz at math, and has a good vocabulary. She's a nice girl, too. That's why they hate to keep reporting to Katie's parents that their daughter can be disruptive in class because she can't stay on task during a group activity or that the teacher has to keep reminding her during quiet reading time to get back to the book and stop rummaging around in her desk, fiddling with her shoelaces, or whispering to her neighbors. Katie's teachers have suggested more than once that it might help if her parents tried to impress upon her the importance of following directions and sticking to assigned activities. At this point her parents can only reply sheepishly that they've tried every way they know to get through to their daughter and that Katie sincerely promises to try but then can't seem to hold on to her vow any more than she can follow through on cleaning her room or setting the table.

Katie's parents are at their wits' end, and their daughter is at risk of falling behind at school. How can someone so smart be so scattered?

As we mentioned in the Introduction, kids who are smart often end up scattered because they lack the brain-based skills we all need to plan and direct activities and to regulate behavior. It's not that they have any problem receiving and organizing the input they get from their senses—what we might ordinarily consider "intelligence." When it comes to smarts, they've got plenty. This is why they may have little trouble comprehending division or fractions or learning how to spell. The trouble shows up when they need to organize output—deciding what to do when and then controlling their own behavior to get there. Because they have what it takes to absorb information and learn math and language and other school subjects, you may assume that much simpler tasks like making a bed or taking turns should be a no-brainer. But that's not the case because your child may have intelligence but lack the executive skills to put it to best use.

What Are Executive Skills?

Let's correct one possible misunderstanding right off the bat. When people hear the term *executive skills*, they assume it refers to the set of skills required of good business executives—skills like financial management, communication, strategic planning, and decision making. There *is* some overlap—executive skills definitely include decision making, planning, and management of all kinds of data, and like the skills used by a business executive, executive skills help kids get done what needs to get done—but in fact the term *executive skills* comes from the neurosciences literature and refers to the brain-based skills that are required for humans to *execute*, or perform, tasks.

Your child (like you) needs executive skills to formulate even the most fundamental plan to initiate a task. For something as simple as getting a glass of milk from the kitchen, he needs to decide to get up and go into the kitchen when he's thirsty, get a glass from the cabinet, put it down on the counter, open the refrigerator and retrieve the milk, close the refrigerator, pour the milk, return the milk to the refrigerator, and then drink it either on the spot or back in the family room where he started out. To carry out this simple task he has to resist the impulse to grab and eat the chips he spots in the cabinet first—they'll only make him thirstier—and to choose a sugar-loaded soda instead of milk. If he finds none of the usual glasses in the cabinet, he has to think to check the dishwasher instead of opting for one of his parents' best crystal goblets. When he finds the milk is almost gone, he has to soothe his own frustration and resist starting a fight with his little sister when he's sure she drank most of the milk. And he has to be sure not to leave a milk ring on the coffee table if he doesn't want to be banned from having his snacks in the family room in the future.

A child with executive skill weaknesses may be able to get a glass of milk without trouble—or he may get distracted, make poor choices, and demonstrate little emotional or behavioral control, leaving the fridge wide open, leaving a trail of milk droplets across the counter and the floor, leaving the milk out on the counter to spoil, and leaving his little sister in tears. But even if he can get himself a glass of milk without incident, you can bet that he will have trouble with the tasks in his life that are more complicated and more demanding of his ability to plan, sustain attention, organize, and regulate his feelings and how he acts on them.

Executive skills are, in fact, what your child needs to make any of your hopes and dreams for his future—or his own hopes and dreams—come true. By late adolescence, our children must meet one fundamental condition: They must function with a reasonable degree of independence. That does not mean that they don't ask for help or seek advice at times. But it does mean that they no longer rely on us to plan or organize their day for them, tell them when to start tasks, bring them items when they forget them, or remind them to pay attention at school. When our children reach this point, our parenting role is coming to an end. We speak of our children as being "on their own," accept this at some level of comfort, and hope for the best for them. Social institutions do the same, defining them as "adult" for most legal purposes.

To reach this stage of independence, the child must develop executive skills. You've probably seen an infant watch his mother leave the room, wait for a short time, and then begin to cry for his mother's return. Or maybe you've listened to your 3-year-old tell herself, in a voice that sounds suspiciously like your own, not to do something. Or how about watching the 9-year-old who actually stops and looks before he races into the street after a ball? In all these cases you're witnessing the development of executive skills.

Our Model

Our initial work in executive skills dates to the 1980s. In evaluating and treating children with traumatic brain injuries, we saw that the source of many cognitive and behavioral difficulties was deficits in executive skills. Although less severe, we noted similar types of problems in children with significant attention disorders. From these origins, we began investigating the development of executive skills for a broad range of children. While there are other systems of executive skills (the Resource section includes references for these systems), our model has been designed to achieve a specific goal: to help us come up with ways that parents and teachers can promote the development of executive skills in kids who have demonstrated weaknesses.

We've based our model on two premises:

1. *Most individuals have an array of executive skill strengths as well as executive skill weaknesses.* In fact, we've found that there seem to be common profiles of strengths and weaknesses. Kids (and adults) who are strong in some specific skills are often weak in other particular skills, and the patterns are predictable. We wanted a model that would enable people to identify those patterns so that kids could be encouraged to draw on their strengths and work to enhance or bypass their weaknesses to improve overall functioning. We also found that it made sense to help parents identify their own strengths and weaknesses so they could be of the greatest help to their kids.

2. *The primary purpose of identifying areas of weakness is to be able to design and implement interventions to address those weaknesses.* We wanted to be able to help chil-

dren build the skills they need or manipulate the environment to minimize or prevent the problems associated with the skill weaknesses. The more discrete the skills are, the easier it is to develop operational definitions of them. When the skills can be operationalized, it's easier to create interventions to improve those operations. For example, let's take the term *scattered*. It's great for a book title because as a parent you read the word and know immediately that it describes your child. But *scattered* could mean forgetful or disorganized, lacking persistence, or distracted. Each one of those problems suggests a different solution. The more specific we can be in our problem definition, the more likely we are to come up with a strategy that actually solves the problem.

The scheme we arrived at consists of 11 skills:

- Response inhibition
- Working memory
- Emotional control
- Sustained attention
- Task initiation
- Planning/prioritization
- Organization
- Time management
- Goal-directed persistence
- Flexibility
- Metacognition

These skills can be organized in two different ways, developmentally (the order in which they develop in kids) and functionally (what they help the child do). Knowing the order in which the skills emerge during infancy, toddlerhood, and beyond, as mentioned earlier, helps you and your child's teachers understand what to expect from a child at a particular age. In a workshop we conducted several years ago with teachers in kindergarten through grade 8, we asked teachers to identify those two or three executive skills in their students that were of greatest concern to them. Teachers in the lower elementary grades focused on task initiation and sustained attention, while middle school teachers stressed time management, organization, and planning/prioritization. Interestingly enough, teachers at all levels selected response inhibition as a skill that they saw lacking in many of their students! The main point, though, is that if you know the order in which skills are expected to develop, you won't end up wasting your time trying to bolster a skill in your 7-year-old that is typically not mastered before age 11. You have enough battles already, you don't need to add beating your head against a brick wall.

The table on pages 16–17 lists the skills in order of emergence, defines each skill, and provides examples of what the skill looks like in younger and older children.

Developmental Progression of Executive Skills

Executive skill	Definition	Examples
Response inhibition	The capacity to think before you act—this ability to resist the urge to say or do something allows your child the time to evaluate a situation and how his or her behavior might impact it.	A young child can wait for a short period without being disruptive. An adolescent can accept a referee's call without an argument.
Working memory	The ability to hold information in memory while performing complex tasks. It incorporates the ability to draw on past learning or experience to apply to the situation at hand or to project into the future.	A young child can hold in mind and follow one- or two-step directions. The middle school child can remember the expectations of multiple teachers.
Emotional control	The ability to manage emotions to achieve goals, complete tasks, or control and direct behavior.	A young child with this skill can recover from a disappointment in a short time. A teenager can manage the anxiety of a game or test and still perform.
Sustained attention	The capacity to keep paying attention to a situation or task in spite of distractibility, fatigue, or boredom.	Completing a 5-minute chore with occasional supervision is an example of sustained attention in the younger child. A teenager can pay attention to homework, with short breaks, for 1 to 2 hours.
Task initiation	The ability to begin projects without undue procrastination, in an efficient or timely fashion.	A young child is able to start a chore or assignment right after instructions are given. A teenager does not wait until the last minute to begin a project.
Planning/ prioritization	The ability to create a roadmap to reach a goal or to complete a task. It also involves being able to make decisions about what's important to focus on and what's not important.	A young child, with coaching, can think of options to settle a peer conflict. A teenager can formulate a plan to get a job.
Organization	The ability to create and maintain systems to keep track of information or materials.	A young child can, with a reminder, put toys in a designated place. A teenager can organize and locate sports equipment.

Executive skill	Definition	Examples
Time management	The capacity to estimate how much time one has, how to allocate it, and how to stay within time limits and deadlines. It also involves a sense that time is important.	A young child can complete a short job within a time limit set by an adult. A teenager can establish a schedule to meet task deadlines.
Goal-directed persistence	The capacity to have a goal, follow through to the completion of the goal, and not be put off by or distracted by competing interests.	A first grader can complete a job to get to recess. A teenager can earn and save money over time to buy something of importance.
Flexibility	The ability to revise plans in the face of obstacles, setbacks, new information, or mistakes. It relates to an adaptability to changing conditions.	A young child can adjust to a change in plans without major distress. A teenager can accept an alternative such as a different job when the first choice is not available.
Metacognition	The ability to stand back and take a bird's-eye view of yourself in a situation, to observe how you problem solve. It also includes self-monitoring and self-evaluative skills (e.g., asking yourself, "How am I doing?" or "How did I do?").	A young child can change behavior in response to feedback from an adult. A teenager can monitor and critique her performance and improve it by observing others who are more skilled.

Infant research tells us that response inhibition, working memory, emotional control, and attention all develop early, in the first 6 to 12 months of life. We see the beginnings of planning when the child finds a way to get a desired object. This is more evident when the child walks. Flexibility shows in the child's reaction to change and can be seen between 12 and 24 months. The other skills, such as task initiation, organization, time management, and goal-directed persistence, come later, ranging from preschool to early elementary school.

Knowing how each skill functions—whether it contributes to your child's thinking or doing—tells you whether the goal of your intervention is to help your child *think* differently or to help your child *behave* differently. If your child has a weak working memory, for instance, you will be working to give the child strategies to help her retrieve critical information (such as what she has to bring home from school for homework) more reliably. If your child has weak emotional control, you will be working to help him use words rather than fists when he discovers that his little brother sat on his model airplane. In fact, though, thinking and doing go hand in hand. Very often, we're teaching kids how to use their thoughts to control their behaviors.

The *thinking skills* are designed to select and achieve goals or to develop solutions to problems. They help children create a picture of a goal and a path to that goal, and they give them the resources they'll need to access along the way to achieve the goal. They also help your child remember the picture, even though the goal may be far away and other events come along to occupy the child's attention and take up space in his or her memory. But to reach the goal, your child needs to use the second set of skills, ones that enable the child *to do* what he needs to do to accomplish the tasks he has set for himself. The second set of skills incorporates *behaviors* that guide the child's actions as he moves along the path.

This organizing scheme is depicted in the table below.

When all goes as planned, beginning in early childhood, we come up with ideas for things we want or need to do, plan or organize the task, squelch thoughts or feelings that interfere with our plans, cheer ourselves on, keep the goal in mind even when obstacles, distractions, or temptations arise, change course as the situation requires, and persist with our efforts until the goal is achieved. This may be as time limited as completing a 10-piece puzzle or as extensive as remodeling our house. Whether we're 3 years old or 30, we use the same set of brain-based executive skills to help us reach our goal.

During much of your child's growth, you can see those executive skills improving. You probably remember having to hold your child's hand on the sidewalk constantly at age 2, then recall being able to walk side by side when your daughter was 4, and then letting her cross the street on her own a few years later. At each stage you were aware that your child's executive skills—her ability to be independent—were growing yet were not developed enough for the child to manage her behavior or solve all the problems she faces without guidance. Everything you teach your child reflects your instinctive understanding that you play a role in helping your child develop and refine these executive skills. So, if parents are playing this role, how do some kids end up off track?

Two Dimensions of Executive Skills: Thinking and Doing

Executive skills involving *thinking* (cognition)	Executive skills involving *doing* (behavior)
Working memory	Response inhibition
Planning/prioritization	Emotional control
Organization	Sustained attention
Time management	Task initiation
Metacognition	Goal-directed persistence
	Flexibility

How Executive Skills Develop in the Brain: Biology and Experience

How do children come by executive skills? As is the case with many of the abilities we have, there are two main contributors: biology and experience. In terms of the biological contribution, the potential for executive skills is innate, already hard-wired into the brain at birth. This is similar to the way that language develops. Of course at birth executive skills, like language, exist *only* as potential. This means that the brain has within it the biological equipment for these skills to develop. But there are a number of biological factors that can influence how these skills develop. Major trauma or physical insult to the child's brain, particularly to the frontal lobes, will affect skill development. The genes that the child inherits from you two can also impact these skills. If you don't have good attention or organization skills, chances are your child will have problems in these areas as well. As to the environment, if it's biologically or physically toxic, the likelihood that the child's executive skills will suffer is increased. Environmental "poisons" can include anything from lead exposure to child abuse. However, assuming reasonably normal biological equipment and the absence of genetic or environmental traumas, brain development can proceed as it's supposed to.

Biology: Growth + Pruning = Executive Skills

At birth, a child's brain weighs about 13 ounces. By the late teenage years brain weight has increased to nearly 3 pounds. A number of changes account for this increase. First, there's rapid growth in the number of nerve cells in the brain. These nerve cells must communicate if the child is to think, feel, or act. So they can "talk" to each other, the nerve cells develop branches that allow them to send and receive information from other nerve cells. The growth of these branches, called *axons* and *dendrites*, is especially fast during the infant and toddler years.

Also during these earliest stages of development, a substance known as *myelin* begins to form a fatty sheath around the axons. This process of myelination insulates the branches that carry the nerve signals, making the "conversations" between nerve cells faster and more efficient. Myelination continues well into the late stages of adolescence and early adulthood and is responsible for the development of what is often called the *white matter* of the brain. The white matter consists of bundles of axons that connect different brain regions and allow them to communicate.

Then there's gray matter. There's a reason that this is the term often used as a metaphor for the learning, thinking power of the brain itself. The gray matter is made up of the nerve cells, or neurons, and the connections between them called the *synapses*, and the development of this type of brain matter is a bit more complex.

Five months into pregnancy, the brain of an unborn child is estimated to have about one hundred billion neurons. This is comparable to what the average adult brain has. Early in childhood, the number of synapses in the brain (about a quadrillion) greatly exceeds the number in the adult brain. If development of gray matter continued at this pace, the adult brain would be enormous. Instead, a different phenomenon occurs. The increase in gray matter—neurons and particularly synapses—peaks before age 5 and is followed by a gradual reduction or "pruning" of the neuron connections. The initial increase happens during a period of rapid learning and experience in early childhood. Recent brain research suggests that as this learning and skill development become more efficient, additional increases in gray matter could actually undermine new learning.

Through pruning, the child consolidates mental skills, with the gray matter connections that are not needed or used dropping away. This period of consolidation continues until a second period of significant growth in gray matter that begins around age 11 or 12, the onset of another period recognized as one of rapid learning and development. This increase is again followed by a period of reduction through pruning over the course of adolescence.

Of significance to what we know about the development of executive skills, research shows that this growth spurt prior to adolescence occurs primarily in the frontal lobes. Considering that scientists generally agree that the frontal brain systems play a key role in the development of executive skills, we can safely say that these areas, which include the frontal and prefrontal cortex, along with connections to adjacent areas, make up the brain base for executive skills. It's as if during the preteen years the brain is preparing itself for the development of executive skills and the significant demands that will be made on those executive skills during adolescence.

The diagram on the facing page shows the human brain with the approximate location of major functions, including executive skills, in the prefrontal cortex.

Researchers at the National Institute of Mental Health also suggest that a "use it or lose it" process may be occurring in the frontal lobes during this time. Neural connections that are used are retained, while those that are not exercised are lost. If this is the case, then the practice of executive skills is critical. It means that kids who practice executive skills are not only learning self-management—independence—but in the process developing brain structures that will support their executive skills into later adolescence and adulthood.

Practice is important to acquisition of executive skills for another reason. Researchers who study the brain using fMRI (functional magnetic resonance imaging) have found that when children and teenagers perform tasks that require these skills, they rely on the prefrontal cortex to do all the work rather than distributing the workload to other specialized regions of the brain, such as the amygdala and the insula, two parts of the brain that are activated when making quick decisions that affect safety and survival (the *fight-or-flight* response). Adults, in contrast, can spread out the workload in part because they've had years of practice to develop the neural pathways to make this possible. Activating executive skills takes more conscious effort with children and with teenagers than it does with adults, which may help

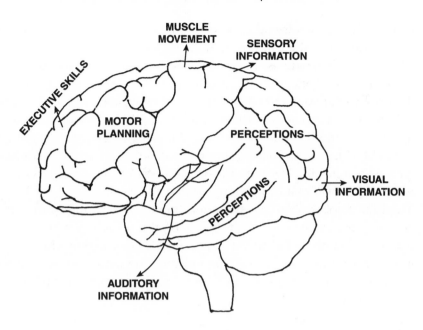

The human brain, with the approximate location of major functions.

explain why they are less inclined to engage their working memory to perform tasks of daily living.

This is where you—and your child's teachers—come in. Clearly childhood offers parents and teachers a critical opportunity to enhance the learning and development of executive skills in a child.

We don't mean to oversimplify. The brain is a very complex organ, and evidence from brain-imaging studies continues to suggest that areas other than the prefrontal cortex are involved in the development of executive skills. But the prefrontal systems are among the last areas of the brain to develop fully, in late adolescence or young adulthood, and are the final, common pathway for managing information and deciding how we will behave. When you consider the critical functions of the frontal lobes, it's easy to see how important these brain structures must be to the development of executive skills:

1. The frontal lobes direct our behavior, helping us decide what we should pay attention to and what actions we should take. *Example:* A 7-year-old sees his brother watching television. He wants to sit and watch with him but decides he should finish his chores first, since he knows his dad will be upset with him if he doesn't.

2. The frontal lobes link our behaviors together so that we can use past experience to guide our behavior and make future decisions. *Example:* A 10-year-old remembers that after she finished cleaning her bedroom last week, her

mom let her have a friend over for pizza. She decides to clean her room in anticipation that she can do the same thing again.

3. The frontal lobes help us control our emotions and our behavior, taking into account external and internal constraints as we work to satisfy our needs and desires. By regulating our emotions and social interactions, the frontal lobes help us meet our needs without causing problems for ourselves or others. *Example:* A mother tells her 6-year-old that he can get a video game at Game Stop, but when they check, the store doesn't have the game he wants. Although angry, he does not tantrum in the store, and he settles for a promise that they will call other stores to find the game.

4. The frontal lobes observe, assess, and fine tune, allowing us to correct our behavior or choose a new strategy based on feedback. *Example:* A 12-year-old misses out on a class field trip because he was the only child in his class who forgot his permission slip. He remembers to get his slip signed the next time, and he makes sure it's in his backpack the night before it has to be handed in at school.

So, where does biology leave your child? First, we know that executive skills are critical to independent living, a basic goal that we assume all parents have for their children. Second, at birth, executive skills exist only as potential; the newborn has no actual executive skills. Third, the frontal lobes, and therefore executive skills, will require 18 to 20 years, or even longer, to develop fully. Given these factors, children cannot rely solely on their own frontal lobes to regulate behavior. What's the solution? We lend them our frontal lobes. Although we may not think of it in these terms, parenting is, among other things, a process of providing executive skill support and coaching for our children.

Experience: Lending Your Child Your Frontal Lobes

In the earliest stages of your child's life, you simply *are* the frontal lobes for your child, and your child has little to contribute. You plan and organize your child's environment so it's safe and comfortable, monitor your child's condition (sleeping, diet), initiate interactions, and problem solve when your child is distressed. As a newborn your child has very few behaviors—pretty much just crying and sleeping—with which to manage her world, and she lives completely in the present. At about 5 or 6 months, however, your infant begins to develop some of the skills that will eventually lead to independence. You may notice your baby's increased awareness, although these early changes are not readily seen by just observing. For the baby, however, the changes are powerful.

One of the new skills to develop at around 5 to 6 months is working memory. Before having this skill, the baby could respond only to what she could see, hear, touch, or taste, right now, in this place right here. But once she can remember people, events, or objects, even for short periods of time, your baby's world gets bigger, and she can have it with her whenever she's awake. She can begin to make choices and "decisions." For example, if Mom leaves and does not come back immediately, the baby can look to the last place she saw her and cry. Mom might return. If this happens, the baby "understands" at some level that "if Mom leaves and I want her back, she'll come if I cry."

As information and experience grow, working memory allows the child to recall a past event, apply it to a present situation, and predict what might happen. For example, suppose your child is now 11 years old. She might say to herself, "Last Saturday after I helped with the laundry, Mom and I had time to go to the pool. I'll ask her if we can do that again after I help her with chores today." Or the 17-year-old could say, "If my boss asks me to work tomorrow night, I need to say I can't. The last time I worked before a test I didn't leave enough time to study and got a lousy grade."

Obviously the baby's recall of Mom is a far cry from her skills at age 11 or 17. But, in her ability to hold a picture of Mom in mind, we can see the beginning of this control. To help her develop a skill like working memory, you can provide your child with certain types of experiences. For an infant, you might provide manipulative, "cause–effect" toys such that when the baby performs an action, like banging it, the toy does something, like move or make a noise. Or you can make a toy "disappear" and have your baby look for it. Once the child can move, you might have her retrieve or search for objects. As she gains language, your child can begin to manage her behavior by remembering directions and rules repeated and displayed by you. And then later again, you can ask questions like "What do you need for this activity?" or "What did you do the last time this happened?"

Obviously, in the early stages of helping a child with this skill, you do most of the work. This includes providing the toys the baby will play with and structuring the games and activities she engages in. Once your child is more mobile and can speak, she is less dependent on you and you don't have to be so close by. In fact, by incorporating some of your actions and words into working memory, she has begun to internalize some of your executive skills!

This brings us to a second key skill that begins developing in the infant at around the same time as working memory: response inhibition. The ability to respond or not respond to a person or an event is at the heart of regulating behavior. We are all aware of the trouble our children can and do get into when they act before thinking. And we are impressed by the self-control of the child who can see a tempting object and not immediately touch or take it.

As with working memory, when an infant begins to develop this skill at around 6 months, we don't see any obvious changes. But between 6 and 12 months, a baby's ability to inhibit a response grows tremendously. You might see your 9-month-old crawling toward her mom in the next room. Whereas a month or two earlier she might have been distracted by finding a favorite toy along the way, now she crawls right past the toy on her way to her mom. During the same period, you may notice that your baby can now withhold some kinds of emotional expression and show others depending on the situation. We've probably all had the experience of trying to engage a baby of this age, who then doesn't respond at all or even turns away. Feels like rejection, doesn't it? Even at this young age, a baby is beginning to learn the powerful effect of responding or not responding to a particular person or situation. The 3- or 4-year-old shows this skill by "using his words" instead of hitting a play-mate who tries to grab his toy. The 9-year-old mentioned a little earlier is using the same response inhibition skill when he looks before running into the street to get a ball. And the 17-year-old shows response inhibition by staying near the speed limit instead of responding to his friend's suggestion, "Let's see what this thing can do."

As parents, we all recognize how critical a skill response inhibition is: Its absence can be dangerous and often leads to conflicts with authority. When your child was a baby, especially once he could creep or crawl, you loaned him this frontal-lobe ability by setting boundaries and limits for him, using gates, doors, and child-proof locks and simply putting a lot of hazardous articles out of reach. You also provided very close supervision. You undoubtedly tried words—a sharp "NO!" or "HOT!"—and in a few cases you may have allowed natural consequences to play a part—or you couldn't prevent them from playing a part, such as when your child suddenly reached out unexpectedly and touched something hot or fell off a couch or cushion. As the child develops, some risks are diminished, such as the stairs once the child has the ability to navigate them safely, but there also are more opportunities.

Besides boundaries and limits, parents also start to teach alternative behaviors (petting the cat instead of pulling its tail, using words instead of hitting). As with working memory, and helped by it, children begin to model parents' behavior and language and make it part of themselves. Depending on what you observe, you start to supervise from a distance, extend the boundaries, use more words, and look to other institutions such as the school to help teach this skill. Since you understand that increased independence and self-management are the goals, you constantly try to balance freedom and supervision. The work you do to lend your children your frontal lobes will, however, always have two components: structuring the environment and directly supervising your child. By observing your behavior, trying to copy it, and doing this repeatedly, your child will begin to learn and take on these skills. Reasonable consistency in the routines and expectations you establish will help. You also will instruct the child using your language. Over time your child will use these words, actually saying them to herself out loud at first, to regulate her own behavior. Over a period of years, with experience, this will become the child's inner voice, heard only by her. We are not meant to be our children's frontal lobes indefinitely. As they develop an inner voice and internalize these skills, our role is naturally decreased.

So, Why Does *Your* Child Lack Certain Executive Skills?

One distinct possibility is a diagnosis of attention-deficit/hyperactivity disorder (ADHD). The prototypical "scattered child" is one with this disorder, and if your child has been diagnosed, you probably already know which of your child's executive skills are most impaired. There is an emerging consensus among researchers that ADHD is fundamentally a disorder of executive skills. Russell Barkley, for example, sees the disorder as one of reduced ability to self-regulate. While a number of executive skills can be affected, response inhibition is key among these and impacts development of the other executive skills. Other researchers emphasize different aspects, but all agree that if a child has ADHD, some executive skills will be impaired. Chief among these are response inhibition, sustained attention, working memory, time management, task initiation, and goal-directed persistence. Others may be affected, but by the time a child reaches adolescence, if he has ADHD, it is likely that parents and teachers will have seen significant weaknesses in this cluster of executive functions. And if a child has this cluster of executive skill weaknesses, it is likely that he has ADHD. Consistent with these findings, emerging brain research suggests that the frontal brain systems of children with ADHD may have differences in physical and chemical makeup that distinguish them from other children. In some of these children, such differences represent a "developmental lag," and over an extended period of time the child (and brain) mature, albeit 2 to 3 years later than in peers. For other children with ADHD, however, this maturation does not take place, and the weaknesses persist until adulthood.

It's important to know that children can and do vary in the development of these and other executive skills without qualifying for a diagnosis of ADHD or any other "clinical" diagnosis. As is the case with almost any set of skills, children (and adults) have strengths and weaknesses that fall along a continuum. There are certainly children for whom time seems irrelevant. And who among us has not known a little "absent-minded professor" who cannot keep track of her belongings? Patterns of strengths and weaknesses like these can be perfectly normal developmental variations. But that doesn't mean you shouldn't do anything about them if they're affecting your child's performance in school, at home, socially, athletically, or in any domain where you naturally want to see your child thrive. Executive skills are increasingly critical for success in our complex world, so if your child resembles Katie from the beginning of this chapter or seems scattered in other ways, it's worth your time—and will ultimately save you time and aggravation—to do what you can to give your child's executive skills a boost.

Kids can be scattered in a variety of ways. Those with ADHD, as well as those with weak organization, working memory, and time management, are very obviously "scattered." They seem lost in time or space, or they lose things in time or space, and they work inefficiently as a result. Some kids, however, are emotionally scattered. Their feelings fracture, sending them off on emotional tangents, blocking their ability to get past obstructions or to problem solve effectively. Or maybe they react so instantaneously and impulsively to what's happening around them that they can't stay on course to get the job done. These children, too, are scattered. They need help corralling or taming their emotions to get on track and get things done.

In the next chapter, you'll be able to assess your own child's executive skill strengths and weaknesses. This is your first step on the path to addressing your child's weaknesses and enhancing his or her strengths.

2

Identifying Your Child's Strengths
and Weaknesses

If you're not accustomed to thinking of your child's growth in terms of executive skills, you might not be fully aware of how much adults do to see that kids learn to make decisions and exercise their gradually developing executive skills. Looking at what schools and teachers do to provide boundaries and room for growth can give you a better overview of how executive skills develop over time.

Think about preschool. A good preschool program imposes a familiar rhythm on the school day that gives children structured group activities as well as the opportunity for free play. Group activities are kept brief because children at this age have short attention spans, and directions are generally given one or two at a time because the kids have a limited ability to hold complex directions or multiple steps in mind. Materials are laid out for children; they're not expected to organize tasks for themselves. While good teachers expect preschool children to help pick up after themselves, they know they have to be there to prompt or cue them to do this.

Free play time gives children the opportunity to practice some executive skills with a little more independence. Here children use planning and organizational skills to make up games and decide on rules. They practice flexibility by taking turns, sharing toys, and allowing another child to be the leader. And the social interactions built into free play enable children to learn to control impulses and manage emotions. These skills are reinforced when preschool teachers give children a few simple rules about behavior (*no running inside; use indoor voices in the classroom*) and review the rules regularly.

By first grade teachers may differentiate between rules for classroom behavior and rules for behavior in other settings like recess, gym, and lunchroom. At this age children are better at modifying their behavior to fit different contexts: it's okay to giggle hysterically with your girlfriends out at recess, for example, but not in the classroom. Teachers also use structure and routines to help children learn to initiate tasks and sustain attention so they can work at them. They do this by prompting children to begin their work at specified times, by giving them tasks that can be completed within a time frame consistent with their attention spans, and by making their expectations clear regarding what the students should accomplish and how long it should take. As the year goes along, they may stretch these skills by gradually increasing the number of tasks that need to be completed and the amount of time each task should take.

Demands on working memory are also greater at this age than in preschool. Teachers assign homework that they expect children to remember, they give them permission slips and ask them to remember to have their parents sign them, and they assume that if children want to eat hot meals in the cafeteria they will remember to bring their lunch money. Of course you help with this too, checking in with your child after school and making sure your child's backpack is packed appropriately before leaving for school.

By late elementary school, teachers begin to work in a more directed fashion on helping children develop organizational and planning skills. Children are expected to keep track of materials, maintain organized notebooks, and keep their desks reasonably neat. Teachers also start assigning long-term projects that require children to follow a sequence of steps and stick to a timeline. Assignments start being more open-ended, which requires students to use metacognition and flexibility to problem solve and consider multiple possible solutions.

Once children reach middle school, the demands on executive skills increase dramatically—and, we would argue, in many cases unrealistically. As we said in Chapter 1, a rapid period of brain development begins at around age 11 or 12—the beginning of middle school in most school systems. In the early stages, development is uneven and unpredictable. That means more support, rather than less, is critical. Think about how children learn to ride a bike. At the point where training wheels are removed, they need more guidance, encouragement, and support from parents than they did when they were riding around with training wheels. The onset of adolescence, and the brain growth that accompanies this stage, requires the same thing.

For most children, middle school is the first time they have multiple teachers, each with his or her own set of expectations regarding how work is to be formatted, notebooks are to be organized, and assignments are handed in. Demands on working memory, planning, organization, and time management increase accordingly. Just take a look at what middle school students are expected to do:

- Remember to write down assignments consistently.
- Keep track of assignments and other materials (notebooks, folders, etc.).
- Know which materials need to be brought home or taken to school daily.

- Plan and monitor long-term assignments, including breaking them down into subtasks and creating timelines.
- Plan how work will be organized and time will be spent, including estimating how much time is required to complete daily assignments as well as long-term assignments.
- Keep track of other responsibilities or belongings—gym clothes, lunch money, permission slips, etc.
- Manage the complexity of changing classes, including the problems associated with having to take different materials to different classes and having teachers with different organizational styles and expectations.

What can parents do about this? It's tempting to pull back on supervision and homework monitoring at this age—in part because children are beginning to look for more independence and freedom from parental scrutiny. While some children's executive skill development allows for a high level of self-management, many are not there yet. You'll know which category your children fall into—but if they fall into the "not there yet" category, then checking in with them daily about homework, helping them keep in mind long-term assignments (for example, by posting them on a calendar located in a prominent place in the house), and asking them how they plan to study for tests, may be advised.

Most teachers don't write their lesson plans specifically with executive skill development in mind. Teachers and parents inherently understand, at least roughly, what they can expect from kids at different ages and set the bar accordingly. Teachers also have had the opportunity for some more formal education in child development. We think, however, that if teachers understood the role executive skills play in fostering independent and self-regulated learning—and how much they are already doing to encourage the development of executive skills—they might do even more. They might teach executive skills explicitly and infuse their instruction with questions and prompts designed to enhance executive skill development. We've written a book, *Executive Skills in Children and Adolescents*, for educators and other professionals such as school psychologists that describes how to do this (see Resources section at the end of the book). And we've just illustrated how standard approaches to education foster executive skill development so that you can begin to see how you can do the same at home—and how you, too, might be able to encourage your child's executive skill development more explicitly.

Think about the daily routines that teachers use to structure the day's activities, the explicit directions they give children, the way they monitor their performance to make sure they understand and follow through on assignments. Think about the way they organize the classroom to make it easy for children to follow those routines. You lead busy lives, and it's unrealistic that you will build your entire day around supervising your child's executive skill development. But if your child seems to be lacking some critical executive skills, you may find it helpful to adapt some strategies teachers use for managing your child at home.

Perhaps even more than teachers, you have an important role to play. This is because there is at least as much demand for executive skills in the home as there is at school. Think about room cleaning, controlling temper, dealing with changes in plans, keeping track of belongings—or any of the other countless examples you will read about in this book. Whereas a teacher has between 20 and 30 students to manage and can't be expected to provide individualized support for every student, the child–parent ratio is more favorable. Think of yourself as your child's tutor when it comes to executive skills. To be a tutor, you don't need to take a course in child development, but you do need to understand what normal executive skill development is and where your child fits along the developmental continuum. That's what this chapter is all about.

How Can You Tell Where Your Child's Executive Skills Are?

There are a number of ways to assess whether your child's development is on target with respect to executive skills.

Is Your Child Generally Meeting Expectations at School?

First of all, if your son or daughter is generally successful in school—earning reasonable grades but also fulfilling the kinds of responsibilities schools demand, such as homework management—chances are his or her executive skills are progressing nicely. Of course there's a chance that your child does fine in school and not as well at home, and that may be why you're reading this book. This can occur for any number of reasons—home is less structured than school, there may be more stressors at home (for example, siblings who get on each other's nerves), or the expectations for executive functioning may be out of sync with your child's development (either too high or too low). Your own executive skill weaknesses could even make home a more challenging place for your child—see Chapter 3 on the goodness of fit between parents and children.

To figure out where your child stands, you need to be aware of the kinds of tasks and responsibilities that are typically expected of children at different ages. The table on page 30 lists the kinds of tasks that require executive skills that children at different ages are usually capable of performing, either on their own or with cueing or supervision from an adult.

How Is Your Child Doing Compared to the Other Kids?

It may be helpful to compare your child to friends or classmates to get a rough estimate of whether executive skills are progressing normally. Keep in mind, though, that there is a *range* of normal development. Just as we don't expect all children to

Developmental Tasks Requiring Executive Skills

Age range	Developmental task
Preschool	Run simple errands (for example, "Get your shoes from the bedroom")
	Tidy bedroom or playroom with assistance
	Perform simple chores and self-help tasks with reminders (for example, clear dishes from table, brush teeth, get dressed)
	Inhibit behaviors: don't touch a hot stove, run into the street, grab a toy from another child, hit, bite, push, etc.
Kindergarten to grade 2	Run errands (two- to three-step directions)
	Tidy bedroom or playroom
	Perform simple chores, self-help tasks; may need reminders (for example, make bed)
	Bring papers to and from school
	Complete homework assignments (20-minute maximum)
	Decide how to spend money (allowance)
	Inhibit behaviors: follow safety rules, don't swear, raise hand before speaking in class, keep hands to self
Grades 3-5	Run errands (may involve time delay or greater distance, such as going to a nearby store or remembering to do something after school)
	Tidy bedroom or playroom (may include vacuuming, dusting, etc.)
	Perform chores that take 15-30 minutes (for example, clean up after dinner, rake leaves)
	Bring books, papers, assignments home and take them back to school
	Keep track of belongings when away from home
	Complete homework assignments (1-hour maximum)
	Plan simple school project such as book reports (select book, read book, write report)
	Keep track of changing daily schedule (for example, different activities after school)
	Save money for desired objects, plan how to earn money
	Inhibit/self-regulate: behave when teacher is out of the classroom; refrain from rude comments, temper tantrums, bad manners
Grades 6-8	Help out with chores around the home, including daily responsibilities and occasional tasks (for example, emptying dishwasher, raking leaves, shoveling snow); tasks may take 60-90 minutes to complete
	Babysit younger siblings or other kids for pay
	Use system for organizing schoolwork, including assignment book, notebooks, etc.
	Follow complex school schedule involving changing teachers and changing schedules
	Plan and carry out long-term projects, including tasks to be accomplished and reasonable timeline to follow; may require planning multiple large projects simultaneously
	Plan time, including after-school activities, homework, family responsibilities; estimate how long it takes to complete individual tasks and adjust schedule to fit
	Inhibit rule breaking in the absence of visible authority

begin walking at 12 months on the dot or combining words at 18 months, it's normal for children to vary around an average point. Some 5-year-olds may be able to remember on their own to brush their teeth after breakfast, but many others do not, and it's not unusual for children at age 8 to need to be reminded to perform this kind of self-care.

If you feel your child might be delayed in terms of executive skill development, you may want to have a conversation with the child's classroom teacher to get another viewpoint from someone who knows your child and can provide some objective feedback. Teachers also have a built-in norm group to compare your child to—especially when they have several years of experience teaching at the same grade level. You may also find it helpful to talk to your child's pediatrician, especially if you think the executive skill weaknesses may be associated with an attention disorder.

Is There a Discernible Pattern to Your Child's Executive Skill Strengths and Weaknesses?

While some children's executive skills are delayed across the board, it's common for children (and for adults, as you'll see in the next chapter) to be stronger in some skills and weaker in others. We've seen certain skill weaknesses (and strengths) appear together in individuals, as mentioned in Chapter 1. Frequently, for instance, children with weak response inhibition also have weak emotional control. These are children who act without thinking and emote without thinking—they're as likely to say something foolish as to fly into a rage at the least provocation. Children who are inflexible also tend to have weak emotional control—a change in plans they weren't expecting leads to a meltdown. Sometimes children are weak in all three executive skills together (response inhibition, emotional control, flexibility): if your child falls into this category, you know how challenging it can be for you to keep your cool when trying to manage the daily trials and tribulations that seem to define your child's life.

Some other combinations we see frequently are these: Youngsters with weak task initiation also often have weak sustained attention—not only are they slow to get started on homework, they also are likely to quit before it's done. These children generally have weak goal-directed persistence. However, we've found that if goal-directed persistence is a relative strength, we can encourage the child to use that skill to override his weaknesses in task initiation and sustained attention. These are the kids we can spur on to get their homework handed in consistently if we tell them that they can earn points for handing in homework on time and, once they have enough points, they can buy that video game they've been hounding us about. Another common combination is time management and planning/prioritization. Kids who have these as strengths seldom have difficulty handling long-term projects. If these are weaknesses, however, they not only don't know where to begin a long-term project, they also don't know *when* to begin it. Finally, we often see a relationship between working memory and organization. Sometimes kids use a strength in one skill to offset a weakness in another (it doesn't matter how messy your bedroom is if you can remember exactly where you put your shinguards)—unfortunately, all too often children who have weak working memory also have weak organizational skills. These are the kids for whom parents need to build in extra time to get ready for soccer games—you'll need it to search through the mess to find the sports equipment!

> Jeremy is 13. He's always been a conscientious student—he keeps his notebooks organized, writes down all his assignments, starts his homework when he gets home from school and doesn't stop until it's done. When given a long-term project, he gets nervous if he doesn't at least start it the day it's assigned. While this all sounds good, managing his nerves is something Jeremy's not particularly good at. If he misplaces a study guide or forgets to bring home a book he needs to use to study for a test the next day, he's likely to have a meltdown. And he just hates creative writing assignments: he can never think of anything to write about, and when he finally gets an idea, he still can't think of what to say beyond the obvious. He asks his mother to help and then is likely to bite her head off if he doesn't like her ideas or if she attempts to get him to do more thinking on his own.
>
> Jeremy's 11-year-old brother Jason has a whole different way of operating. He views homework as a burden to be put off as long as possible and completed as quickly as possible. His backpack is a mess because he just throws in papers and books at the end of the day, thinking he'll sort things out at a later time (that never seems to come). His mother is constantly on his case in the morning about getting ready for school on time and at night about his homework. While the drudgery of daily math and spelling homework drives him nuts, he loves the freedom that more open-ended assignments give him. He has a lively imagination and could talk for hours about how fantasy fiction differs from science fiction. Science projects that require him to figure out how to make something work or work better are so much fun he doesn't even think of them as homework. He can't understand why his brother gets so worked up over things. His brother, on the other hand, hates the way Jeremy keeps their dad waiting every morning as he ambles through his morning routine, oblivious to the fact that they risk being late for school.

Jeremy's best developed executive skills—task initiation, sustained attention, and time management—seem to be his brother's weakest skills. On the other hand, Jason's strengths—flexibility, metacognition, and emotional control—are in short supply for Jeremy. When planning ways to help children, it's helpful to understand how executive skills often form a cluster of strengths and weaknesses. Strategies to

address one weakness often help bolster another. If we can help Jeremy handle difficult situations more flexibly, we may end up helping him manage his emotions more
effectively as well. And if we can improve Jason's ability to begin tedious tasks without undue procrastination, we may find he has more time—or more energy—to finish them.

Using Rating Scales to Find Your Child's Strengths and Weaknesses

By now, you may be familiar enough with the individual executive skills to describe
your own child's strengths and weaknesses pretty accurately. You can confirm your
assessment by completing one of the rating scales on your child. Because well-
developed executive skills look different at different ages, we've created four questionnaires, representing four age groups (preschool, lower elementary, upper elementary, and middle school). Select the scale that fits your child.

While some of the items on these scales are quite explicit (for example, "Can
complete a chore that takes 15–20 minutes"), others will require some judgment on
your part (for example, "Adjusts easily to unplanned-for situations"). When you're
not sure how to rate an item, think about other children the same age as your child,
or think about what an older sibling was like at the same age.

....

EXECUTIVE SKILLS QUESTIONNAIRE FOR CHILDREN—
PRESCHOOL/KINDERGARTEN VERSION

Read each item below and then rate that item based on how well it describes your child. Then add the three scores in each section. Find the three highest and three lowest scores.

Strongly agree	5
Agree	4
Neutral	3
Disagree	2
Strongly disagree	1

Score

1. Acts appropriately in some situations where danger is obvious (e.g., avoiding hot stove).   _____

2. Can share toys without grabbing.   _____

3. Can wait for a short period of time when instructed by an adult.   _____

TOTAL SCORE: _____

4. Runs simple errands (e.g., gets shoes from bedroom when asked).   _____

5. Remembers instructions just given.   _____

6. Follows two steps of a routine with only one prompt per step.   _____

TOTAL SCORE: _____

7. Can recover fairly quickly from a disappointment or change in plans.   _____

8. Is able to use nonphysical solutions when another child takes toy away.   _____

9. Can play in a group without becoming overly excited.   _____

TOTAL SCORE: _____

10. Can complete a 5-minute chore (may need supervision).   _____

11. Can sit through preschool "circle time" (15-20 minutes).   _____

12. Can listen to one to two stories at a sitting.   _____

TOTAL SCORE: _____

13. Will follow an adult directive right after it is given.   _____

14. Will stop playing to follow an adult instruction when directed.   _____

15. Is able to start getting ready for bed at set time with one reminder.   _____

TOTAL SCORE: _____

16. Can finish one task or activity before beginning another.   _____

17. Is able to follow a brief routine or plan developed by someone else (with model or demo).   _____

18. Can complete a simple art project with more than one step.   _____

TOTAL SCORE: _____

(cont.)

From *Smart but Scattered* by Peg Dawson and Richard Guare. Copyright 2009 by The Guilford Press.

19. Hangs up coat in appropriate place (may need one reminder). _____
20. Puts toys in proper locations (with reminders). _____
21. Clears off place setting after eating (may need one reminder). _____

TOTAL SCORE: _____

22. Can complete daily routines without dawdling (with some cues/ reminders). _____
23. Can speed up and finish something more quickly when given a reason to do so. _____
24. Can finish a small chore within time limits (e.g., make bed before turning on TV). _____

TOTAL SCORE: _____

25. Will direct other children in play or pretend play activities. _____
26. Will seek assistance in conflict resolution for a desired item. _____
27. Will try more than one solution to get to a simple goal. _____

TOTAL SCORE: _____

28. Is able to adjust to change in plans or routines (may need warning). _____
29. Recovers quickly from minor disappointments. _____
30. Is willing to share toys with others. _____

TOTAL SCORE: _____

31. Can make minor adjustment in construction project or puzzle when first attempt fails. _____
32. Can find novel (but simple) use of a tool to solve a problem. _____
33. Makes suggestions to another child for how to fix something. _____

TOTAL SCORE: _____

	KEY		
Items	**Executive skill**	**Items**	**Executive skill**
1–3	Response inhibition	4–6	Working memory
7–9	Emotional control	10–12	Sustained attention
13–15	Task initiation	16–18	Planning/prioritization
19–21	Organization	22–24	Time management
25–27	Goal-directed persistence	28–30	Flexibility
31–33	Metacognition		

Your child's executive skill strengths (highest scores)

_____

_____

_____

Your child's executive skill weaknesses (lowest scores)

_____

_____

_____

EXECUTIVE SKILLS QUESTIONNAIRE FOR CHILDREN—LOWER ELEMENTARY VERSION (GRADES 1-3)

Read each item below and then rate that item based on how well it describes your child. Then add the three scores in each section. Find the three highest and three lowest scores.

Strongly agree	5
Agree	4
Neutral	3
Disagree	2
Strongly disagree	1

Score

1. Can follow simple classroom rules. _____
2. Can be in close proximity to another child without need for physical contact. _____
3. Can wait until parent gets off phone before telling him/her something (may need one reminder). _____

TOTAL SCORE: _____

4. Is able to run errand with two to three steps. _____
5. Remembers instructions given a couple of minutes earlier. _____
6. Follows two steps of a routine with one prompt. _____

TOTAL SCORE: _____

7. Can tolerate criticism from an adult. _____
8. Can deal with perceived "unfairness" without undue upset. _____
9. Is able to adjust behavior quickly in new situation (e.g., calming down after recess). _____

TOTAL SCORE: _____

10. Can spend 20-30 minutes on homework assignments. _____
11. Can complete a chore that takes 15-20 minutes. _____
12. Can sit through a meal of normal duration. _____

TOTAL SCORE: _____

13. Can remember and follow simple one- to two-step routines (such as brushing teeth and combing hair after breakfast). _____
14. Can get right to work on classroom assignment following teacher instruction to begin. _____
15. Will start homework at established time (with one reminder). _____

TOTAL SCORE: _____

16. Can carry out a two- to three-step project of own design (e.g., arts and crafts, construction). _____
17. Can figure out how to earn/save money for an inexpensive toy. _____
18. Can carry out two- to three-step homework assignment with support (e.g., book report). _____

TOTAL SCORE: _____

(cont.)

19. Puts coat, winter gear, sports equipment in proper locations (may need reminder). _____
20. Has specific places in bedroom for belongings. _____
21. Doesn't lose permission slips, notices from school. _____

TOTAL SCORE: _____

22. Can complete a short task within time limits set by an adult. _____
23. Can build in appropriate amount of time to complete a chore before a deadline (may need assistance). _____
24. Can complete a morning routine within time limits (may need practice). _____

TOTAL SCORE: _____

25. Will stick with challenging task to achieve desired goal (e.g., building difficult Lego construct). _____
26. Will come back to a task later if interrupted. _____
27. Will work on a desired project for several hours or over several days. _____

TOTAL SCORE: _____

28. Plays well with others (doesn't need to be in charge, can share, etc.). _____
29. Tolerates redirection by teacher when not following instructions. _____
30. Adjusts easily to unplanned-for situations (e.g., substitute teacher). _____

TOTAL SCORE: _____

31. Can adjust behavior in response to feedback from parent or teacher. _____
32. Can watch what happens to others and change behavior accordingly _____
33. Can verbalize more than one solution to a problem and make the best choice. _____

TOTAL SCORE: _____

KEY			
Items	**Executive skill**	**Items**	**Executive skill**
1-3	Response inhibition	4-6	Working memory
7-9	Emotional control	10-12	Sustained attention
13-15	Task initiation	16-18	Planning/prioritization
19-21	Organization	22-24	Time management
25-27	Goal-directed persistence	28-30	Flexibility
31-33	Metacognition		

Your child's executive skill strengths (highest scores)

_____

_____

_____

Your child's executive skill weaknesses (lowest scores)

_____

_____

_____

EXECUTIVE SKILLS QUESTIONNAIRE FOR CHILDREN—
UPPER ELEMENTARY VERSION (GRADES 4-5)

Read each item below and then rate that item based on how well it describes your child. Then add the three scores in each section. Find the three highest and three lowest scores.

Strongly agree	5
Agree	4
Neutral	3
Disagree	2
Strongly disagree	1

Score

1. Handles conflict with peer without getting into physical fight (may lose temper). _____

2. Follows home or school rules in the absence of an adult's immediate presence. _____

3. Can calm down or de-escalate quickly from an emotionally charged situation when prompted by an adult. _____

TOTAL SCORE: _____

4. Remembers to follow a routine chore after school without reminders. _____

5. Brings books, papers, assignments to and from school. _____

6. Keeps track of changing daily schedule (e.g., different activities after school). _____

TOTAL SCORE: _____

7. Doesn't overreact to losing a game or not being selected for an award. _____

8. Can accept not getting what he/she wants when working/playing in a group. _____

9. Acts with restraint in response to teasing. _____

TOTAL SCORE: _____

10. Can spend 30-60 minutes on homework assignments. _____

11. Can complete a chore that takes 30-60 minutes (may need a break). _____

12. Is able to attend sports practice, church service, etc., for 60-90 minutes. _____

TOTAL SCORE: _____

13. Is able to follow a three- to four-step routine that has been practiced. _____

14. Can complete three to four classroom assignments in a row. _____

(cont.)

15. Can follow established homework schedule (may need reminder to get started). _____

TOTAL SCORE: _____

16. Can make plans to do something special with a friend (e.g., go to movies). _____

17. Can figure out how to earn/save money for a more expensive purchase. _____

18. Can carry out long-term project for school, with most steps broken down by someone else. _____

TOTAL SCORE: _____

19. Can put belongings in appropriate places in bedroom or other locations in house. _____

20. Brings in toys from outdoors after use or at end of day (may need reminder). _____

21. Keeps track of homework materials and assignments. _____

TOTAL SCORE: _____

22. Can complete daily routines within reasonable time limits without assistance. _____

23. Can adjust homework schedule to allow for other activities (e.g., starting early if there's an evening Scout meeting). _____

24. Is able to start long-term projects enough in advance to reduce time crunch (may need help with this). _____

TOTAL SCORE: _____

25. Can save allowance for 3-4 weeks to make a desired purchase. _____

26. Is able to follow a practice schedule to get better at a desired skill (sport, instrument)—may need reminders. _____

27. Can maintain a hobby over several months. _____

TOTAL SCORE: _____

28. Doesn't "get stuck" on things (e.g., disappointments, slights). _____

29. Can "shift gears" when plans have to change due to unforeseen circumstances. _____

30. Can do "open-ended" homework assignments (may need assistance). _____

TOTAL SCORE: _____

31. Is able to anticipate in advance the result of a course of action and make adjustments accordingly (e.g., to avoid getting in trouble). _____

32. Can articulate several solutions to problems and explain the best one. _____

33. Enjoys the problem-solving component of school assignment or video games. _____

TOTAL SCORE: _____

(cont.)

	KEY		
Items	**Executive skill**	**Items**	**Executive skill**
1-3	Response inhibition	4-6	Working memory
7-9	Emotional control	10-12	Sustained attention
13-15	Task initiation	16-18	Planning/prioritization
19-21	Organization	22-24	Time management
25-27	Goal-directed persistence	28-30	Flexibility
31-33	Metacognition		

Your child's executive skill strengths (highest scores)

_____

_____

_____

Your child's executive skill weaknesses (lowest scores)

_____

_____

_____

Read each item below and then rate that item based on how well it describes your child. Then add the three scores in each section. Find the three highest and three lowest scores.

Strongly agree	5
Agree	4
Neutral	3
Disagree	2
Strongly disagree	1

Score

1. Is able to walk away from confrontation or provocation by a peer. ____

2. Can say no to a fun activity if other plans have already been made. ____

3. Resists saying hurtful things when with a group of friends. ____

TOTAL SCORE: _____

4. Able to keep track of assignments and classroom rules of multiple teachers. ____

5. Remembers events or responsibilities that deviate from the norm (e.g., special instructions for field trips, extracurricular activities). ____

6. Remembers multistep directions, given sufficient time and practice. ____

TOTAL SCORE: _____

7. Is able to "read" reactions from friends and adjust behavior accordingly. ____

8. Can accept not getting what he/she wants when working/playing in a group. ____

9. Can be appropriately assertive (e.g., asking teacher for help, inviting someone to dance at a school dance). ____

TOTAL SCORE: _____

10. Can spend 60-90 minutes on homework (may need one or more breaks). ____

11. Can tolerate family gatherings without complaining of boredom or getting in trouble. ____

12. Can complete chores that take up to 2 hours (may need breaks). ____

TOTAL SCORE: _____

(cont.)

13. Can make and follow nightly homework schedule without undue procrastination. _____

14. Can start chores at agreed-on time (e.g., right after school; may need written reminder). _____

15. Can set aside fun activity when he/she remembers a promised obligation. _____

TOTAL SCORE: _____

16. Can do research on the Internet either for school or to learn something of interest. _____

17. Can make plans for extracurricular activities or summertime activities. _____

18. Can carry out a long-term project for school with little or no support from adults. _____

TOTAL SCORE: _____

19. Can maintain notebooks as required for school. _____

20. Doesn't lose sports equipment/personal electronics. _____

21. Keeps study area at home reasonably tidy. _____

TOTAL SCORE: _____

22. Can usually finish homework before bedtime. _____

23. Can make good decisions about priorities when time is limited (e.g., coming home from school to finish project rather than playing with friends). _____

24. Can spread out a long-term project over several days. _____

TOTAL SCORE: _____

25. Is able to increase effort to improve performance (e.g., change study strategies to earn a higher grade on a test or bring up report card grades). _____

26. Willing to engage in effortful tasks to earn money. _____

27. Willing to practice without reminders to improve a skill. _____

TOTAL SCORE: _____

28. Is able to adjust to different teachers, classroom rules, and routines. _____

29. Is willing to adjust in a group situation when a peer is behaving inflexibly. _____

30. Is willing to adjust to or accept a younger sibling's agenda (e.g., allowing someone else to select a family movie). _____

TOTAL SCORE: _____

(cont.)

31. Can accurately evaluate own performance (e.g., in sports event or school performance). ____

32. Is able to see impact of behavior on peers and make adjustments (e.g., to fit in with a group or avoid being teased). ____

33. Can perform tasks requiring more abstract reasoning. ____

TOTAL SCORE: _____

KEY			
Items	**Executive skill**	**Items**	**Executive skill**
1-3	Response inhibition	4-6	Working memory
7-9	Emotional control	10-12	Sustained attention
13-15	Task initiation	16-18	Planning/prioritization
19-21	Organization	22-24	Time management
25-27	Goal-directed persistence	28-30	Flexibility
31-33	Metacognition		

Your child's executive skill strengths (highest scores)	**Your child's executive skill weaknesses (lowest scores)**
_____	_____
_____	_____
_____	_____

Capitalizing on Strengths

How can you use this information to help your child? Look at your child's executive skill strengths. These should be skills that you can take advantage of to help him or her function effectively in daily activities. We gave you an example earlier of using goal-directed persistence to override problems with task initiation and sustained attention. Another example would be using your child's metacognitive strengths to help him solve problems that arise from weaknesses in other executive skills ("Dan, I know you're good at solving problems—what's something we could do to help you keep track of your sports equipment so you don't have to run around like a madman before every game?"). You can also build on your child's executive skill strengths by communicating that she is particularly good at this skill and reinforcing her for using it effectively. For instance, if your daughter is pretty good at task initiation, she can become even better if she is praised for using this skill. "I like the way you get started on homework before dinner," you might tell her, or "I like it that I don't have to tell you more than once when it's time to feed your rabbits."

Perhaps your child's strongest skills are still not particularly effective (an average score of 9 or less would suggest this is the case). Nonetheless, you can build on this skill by noting those times when your child does manage to use the skill effectively and praise him for doing so. If response inhibition falls a little short, then praising your son for "holding his fire" when his younger brother messed up his Lego creation may help him improve this skill.

Praising children for using executive skills need not be reserved for the areas of comparative strength. *Any time* you see your child making good use of any skill, the effective use of praise can help build that skill. This may be the most underused strategy that parents and teachers have to help children build skills and appropriate behavior. We will discuss this in greater detail in Chapter 8.

Addressing Weaknesses

Now look at your child's executive skill weaknesses. Chances are, when you think about the kinds of things your child does that gets him in trouble or gets you particularly annoyed, they fall into one of these three domains. Maybe it drives you nuts that your son consistently forgets to bring home the books he needs for homework or leaves expensive sports equipment on the playing field or at his friend's house. It's likely that working memory is one of his areas of weakness. If your daughter's messy bedroom is a bone of contention between you, and if it seems like she's always frantically looking through her backpack for missing papers or study guides, then organization is likely a significant challenge for her.

So what do you do about these areas of weakness? Part III of the book will take up each executive skill in turn and outline intervention strategies that can either minimize the negative impact of the weakness or help children improve their ability to use the skill. You may be tempted to jump ahead and read the chapters that address your child's weakness—especially if you have problems with response inhibition yourself, something we'll help you discover in the next chapter. However, we encourage you to read through all the chapters in this book in order before getting down to work because we lay a foundation that we think will help you identify the most effective interventions given your child's developmental level and the nature of his or her difficulties. Before you get to Part III, we have a little more information to offer on what you're dealing with and then, in Part II, some important general advice.

3

··

How Your Own Executive Skill Strengths and Weaknesses Matter

It's 8:30 in the morning, and Donna's 14-year-old son, Jim, left for school over an hour ago. Now it's time for Donna to get to work, but when she checks to make sure her cell phone is in her purse, she finds it's missing. She remembers that Jim borrowed it yesterday when he was at a baseball game with a friend and used it to call her for a ride home. Would he have put it in his sports bag, his jacket, or his jeans after he called her? This is why she finds herself in his bedroom rummaging through the rubble for any sign of her phone. Usually she just closes the door to his room so she doesn't have to look at the mess. This is her latest strategy for coping with this problem that has caused tension in their relationship for years. Donna, according to her son, is a "neat freak"—someone who won't leave a single dirty dish in the sink, who hates it when her kids leave the top off the toothpaste tube, and who stacks magazines neatly on the coffee table in the living room, carefully recycling any issues more than a month old. Jim, in his mother's words, is a "total slob"—it would never occur to him to throw out old candy wrappers, let alone keep important things like cell phones in a dependable place. Chances are he knows exactly where it is, but she has no way of contacting him. With a cursory glance at the mess in his bedroom, Donna gives up. She hopes there's no emergency when she's on the road at work for which she'll regret not having her phone.

Ten-year-old Mindy's dance practice ended 25 minutes ago, and all the rest of the students have been picked up by their parents and are on their way home while her father is nowhere to be seen. Mindy paces back and forth in the hall outside the classroom, looking out the window and stopping to check each time a car enters the busy community center parking lot, hoping it's her father. Her fists are clenched and her face looks like a storm cloud. When it's her mother's turn to pick her up, she can count on her being early. She and her mom are time conscious. Mindy gets ready for school with at least 15 minutes to spare before she has to go to the bus stop. She knows exactly how long it will take her to do her homework, and she makes sure she finishes it before dinner every night. Her dad, though, seems to have no notion of time. He's chronically late, always tries to do "just one more thing" before leaving for work in the morning or shutting his office door at night. And if he gets stopped on the way to his car by a colleague with a question after work . . . well, forget it, that's a 10-minute conversation at least, even if he knows he's promised his wife he'll be home at a certain time. Whenever her dad's late, Mindy always starts imagining something bad happening to him. Maybe he got in a car accident on the way over—or maybe he forgot about her and scheduled a late afternoon meeting! When she sees her dad's car pull up right outside the community center, she's out the door before he can open the car door. "Where were you?!" she says, an edge of panic in her voice. "Hey," her dad says, stepping out of the car and taking her in his arms. "You knew I wouldn't forget you," he says soothingly. "I just had a phone call that went on longer than I thought it would."

Sound familiar? If your son's or daughter's executive skill weaknesses drive you crazy, there's a good chance that it's because you're strong in those executive skills. You probably know how this goes just like Donna does: Your son needs to be prodded repeatedly to get ready for school on time; you haven't been late to work in 5 years. Your daughter plunges into histrionics at the slightest change in plans; you like nothing better than to be surprised. Your child never seems to start his homework without being threatened with the loss of every privilege he has or to finish it unless you're standing over him throughout; you always get your chores and errands out of the way first thing so they're not hanging over your head. Donna can't fathom how her son can stand to be so disorganized. But that's because she doesn't have the strong working memory that Jim relies on and doesn't understand how it can substitute to a great degree for the organizational skills that he lacks. Likewise, if you believe in starting unpleasant tasks right away and seem to know instinctively how to break down a large task into smaller subtasks, it may be doubly irritating to see your son put off long-term projects until the last minute and then not have any idea what to do first.

In our work with children with executive skill problems, we've found that the problems often seem more severe when those children have parents with a very different pattern of strengths and weaknesses. If Donna lacked organizational skills too, she might empathize with her son's deficiencies and more readily share how she has learned to compensate for them. Instead she sometimes feels her son must have come from another planet, and it's hard for her to bridge this gap and help him build the skills he lacks.

Mindy can't imagine why her dad doesn't see the importance of being on time, and she can't easily calm herself when his tardiness upsets her. Because he doesn't think being a little late is a big deal and rarely loses his cool, Mindy's father keeps showing up late to pick her up and keeps marveling at how she "overreacts." The two don't really understand each other, and Mindy's weakness in emotional control isn't addressed—at least not by her father.

When parents have one set of executive skill strengths and weaknesses and their children have another set, they're missing out on what we call "goodness of fit." Not only is the potential for conflict between parent and child over daily routines increased, but the stage isn't set for helping the child build the deficient skills. As you'll learn in Chapters 5–8, and then once you get into the interventions described in Part III, there are various ways that you can help a child compensate for and even eliminate weaknesses in executive skills. They all, to some degree, involve interacting differently with your child. Until you understand how your executive skill strengths and weaknesses dovetail—or don't—with your child's, it will be tough to know where to change your act. When you have a clearer understanding, about the nature of executive skills in general and about your own processing style specifically, you'll find it easier to understand your child and to identify intervention strategies that are a good match for your child's strengths.

Ironically, it's not just having the same strengths that helps you and your child work together toward getting things done effectively and helping the child practice executive skills to further her development. It can also be having the same weaknesses. But only if you're aware of this fit. If you really don't start from the understanding that you both lack, say, the ability to sustain attention, you can end up terribly frustrated when you try to complete a big chore, like cleaning out the garage, together. A lot of blame can be flung back and forth as you both face the fact that an unpleasant task is being dragged out longer and longer. It's easier to see that your child isn't paying attention than it is to see the same weakness in yourself. This is why it's so important to identify your own executive skill strengths and weaknesses in this chapter. When you go into projects and routines knowing that you and your child face the same challenges, you can find ways to work through them together with humor and cooperation.

When you discover your own executive skill patterns, you might also find another way that you and your child actually have goodness of fit that you wouldn't expect. You may have a strength that is a natural complement to your child's weakness. Mindy's dad, for example, is highly flexible. Once he recognizes this as a strength, he might be able to strategize how he could show Mindy that flexibility can help her deal with situations where her expectations aren't going to be met. Maybe she can learn that there are options that would prevent her from simply getting upset and out of control. For example, he might explain that he is not as good at keeping track of time as she is and that she should build in an extra 20–30 minutes before she starts worrying about him. Or he might suggest they make a game of estimating how late he will be—she could write down her estimate on a piece of paper, and if it matches the time he arrives, she earns a gold star. Both these ideas have the added benefit of helping Mindy understand that she and her father are different. Life is full of people being late, and if Mindy can learn to accept her father's tardiness—who knows?—it may help her be tolerant of her husband when she finds she married someone just like "dear old Dad."

To help you understand your own executive skill strengths and weaknesses, take the brief questionnaire that follows.

....

EXECUTIVE SKILLS QUESTIONNAIRE FOR PARENTS

Read each item and then rate how well you think it describes you. Then add the three scores in each section.

Strongly disagree	1
Disagree	2
Tend to disagree	3
Neutral	4
Tend to agree	5
Agree	6
Strongly agree	7

Your score

1. I don't jump to conclusions. _____
2. I think before I speak. _____
3. I don't take action without having all the facts. _____

YOUR TOTAL SCORE: _____

4. I have a good memory for facts, dates, and details. _____
5. I am very good at remembering the things I have committed to do. _____
6. I seldom need reminders to complete tasks. _____

YOUR TOTAL SCORE: _____

7. My emotions seldom get in the way when performing on the job. _____
8. Little things do not affect me emotionally or distract me from the task at hand. _____
9. I can defer my personal feelings until after a task has been completed. _____

YOUR TOTAL SCORE: _____

10. No matter what the task, I believe in getting started as soon as possible. _____
11. Procrastination is usually not a problem for me. _____
12. I seldom leave tasks to the last minute. _____

YOUR TOTAL SCORE: _____

13. I find it easy to stay focused on my work. _____
14. Once I start an assignment, I work diligently until it's completed. _____
15. Even when interrupted, I find it easy to get back and complete the job at hand. _____

YOUR TOTAL SCORE: _____

16. When I plan out my day, I identify priorities and stick to them. _____
17. When I have a lot to do, I can easily focus on the most important things. _____

(cont.)

18. I typically break big tasks down into subtasks and timelines. _____

YOUR TOTAL SCORE: _____

19. I am an organized person. _____

20. It is natural for me to keep my work area neat and organized. _____

21. I am good at maintaining systems for organizing my work. _____

YOUR TOTAL SCORE: _____

22. At the end of the day, I've usually finished what I set out to do. _____

23. I am good at estimating how long it takes to do something. _____

24. I am usually on time for appointments and activities. _____

YOUR TOTAL SCORE: _____

25. I think of myself as being driven to meet my goals. _____

26. I easily give up immediate pleasures to work on long-term goals. _____

27. I believe in setting and achieving high levels of performance. _____

YOUR TOTAL SCORE: _____

28. I routinely evaluate my performance and devise methods for personal improvement. _____

29. I am able to step back from a situation to make objective decisions. _____

30. I "read" situations well and can adjust my behavior based on the reactions of others. _____

YOUR TOTAL SCORE: _____

31. I take unexpected events in stride. _____

32. I easily adjust to changes in plans and priorities. _____

33. I consider myself flexible and adaptive to change. _____

YOUR TOTAL SCORE: _____

KEY			
Items	Executive skill	Items	Executive skill
1–3	Response inhibition	4–6	Working memory
7–9	Emotional control	10–12	Sustained attention
13–15	Task initiation	16–18	Planning/prioritization
19–21	Organization	22–24	Time management
25–27	Goal-directed persistence	28–30	Metacognition
31–33	Flexibility		

Your executive skill strengths (highest scores)

Your executive skill weaknesses (lowest scores)

_____   _____

_____   _____

_____   _____

Because this is a brief questionnaire and includes a limited number of items for each executive skill, the results may not have captured you perfectly, but they should give you an idea of the executive skills that come most easily to you as well as those with which you struggle the most. From using this questionnaire with groups of adults over the years, we've found that the average score for each of the 12 executive skill domains is 13–15 (out of a maximum of 21 points, and the average difference between the highest domain score and the lowest is about 14 (with the maximum point spread possible being 18). This suggests that while people in general see themselves as having fairly well developed executive skills overall, at the same time, they are generally able to identify distinct strengths and weaknesses.

If you're still not sure about your executive skills profile, go through the strengths and weaknesses one by one and ask yourself whether you remember having the same strengths and weaknesses as a child. If so, these are likely true inherent executive skill strengths and weaknesses. As a child, for instance (this is Peg speaking), I can remember my mother harping on me to clean my room. It wasn't that I didn't like a clean bedroom—it's just that it took *so much effort* to keep my bedroom tidy. Even now, as an adult, I continue to struggle with that. In contrast, I remember always being keenly aware of time—how long it takes to do things, how much time it takes to get someplace—and today I have excellent time management skills. I see the same strengths and weaknesses in my children—both my adult sons struggle with tidiness, but they're always on time for any appointment. However, they seem to have inherited their ability to manage their emotions from their father, and to this day they tease me when I panic over misplaced car keys or other minor or temporary inconveniences.

Of course you may be reminded by this exercise, as one of our workshop participants is occasionally, that where you once had a weakness you now have a

---

Flexibility: The Antidote to a Parent-Child Mismatch

Did your questionnaire scores show a strength in flexibility? If so, you're in luck if you and your child have opposite patterns of executive skills. Flexibility means you're probably pretty adaptable, and that makes you less likely to be irritated or annoyed by your child's executive skill weaknesses, whatever they are.

- Use your awareness of this gift to make a special promise to stay loose in those situations where your child's executive skill weaknesses *do* tend to drive you crazy.
- On the downside, you may find it hard to put in place an intervention to address an area of weakness in your child and stick with it long enough for it to work. But let's stick with the positive for now, OK?

strength—because a parent helped you learn an executive skill by reinforcing it. Reviewing your childhood memories about executive skill strengths and weaknesses and comparing your skills to those of your own parents and those of your children will hone your ability to see how parents and children can have similar or different executive skills. This exercise may help you learn more about yourself but also about the fit between you and your child.

In the case of the second pattern—when your weaknesses coincide with your child's—tensions often arise because your child lacks the capacity to "pick up the slack" or to counteract the negative effect of your own weaknesses. For instance, if you and your daughter have weak working memory and lousy organizational skills, then keeping track of things like field trip permission slips, report cards that need signatures, or soccer shinguards will be very difficult. We might also add that spouses who have different executive skill profiles often run into trouble with each other for the same reasons.

Compensating for a Fit That's Not So Good

So, what to do when these patterns emerge? Here are some tips that might make things go a little more smoothly:

When your strengths coincide with your child's weaknesses:

• *See if you and your child can come to some agreement that your child will accept your help where he's weak and you're strong so his weaknesses don't get him in trouble.* For instance, if you're good at time management and your son is not, he may accept your help in estimating how long it will take to finish writing the first draft of his book report and can plan his time accordingly. We hasten to add, however, that some—perhaps many—children will resist this kind of advice or assistance from their parents, particularly as adolescence kicks in and they have no interest in listening to their parents' advice on *any* matter, let alone something where their parents seem to feel their own skills exceed those of their children.

• *Be creative in using your strengths to help your child enhance her skills.* If you have good organizational skills, for instance, you are more likely to be able to help your child develop effective organizational systems (described in more detail in Chapter 16) than if this is a weakness for you, too. But as we just said, your child may not be that open to this kind of help from you, so you might have to be innovative and subtle about it. Let's say your daughter is highly artistic and visual. You know that having containers that help you organize materials is an easy way to stay on top of regular tasks. Maybe your daughter will be open to using these tools if you take her on a shopping trip to buy bright-colored trays and compartmentalized storage pieces along with stickers and markers for decorating them. As you read earlier, Mindy's dad used his strength in flexibility to come up with a humorous way to help his daughter handle her emotions. A parent who's good at planning might help her child learn how to carry out a complex task by writing down each step on a separate index card, then shuffle the cards and have her child put them in a logical sequence.

• *Make a point of identifying where you are weak and your child is strong.* If you understand that the source of some of your frustration lies in the fact that your skills profile is very different from your child's, you may feel less irritated and frustrated when you see the weakness coming out in your child. But don't stop there; remind yourself—and your child—of where the child has a strength that you lack. This will really keep up morale when you need it most. Perhaps response inhibition is a strength of yours and a weakness of your son's. You may be able to put that in some perspective by acknowledging that flexibility, an equally important executive skill, is a strong suit for your son but not for you: "Remember the last time we went to the movies together and the movie I wanted to see was sold out? I was ready to walk out and go home in a huff, and you just said, 'Hey, maybe there's another movie we can see.' And when it turned out there was nothing we wanted to watch, you were the one who suggested we play a round of miniature golf and get back to the theater really early for the next showing. You bounce back much better than I do!"

When you and your child share the same weaknesses:

• *Work at it so you can laugh about shared weaknesses rather than weep about them.* "Son, you and I are both organizationally challenged," you might say, "so maybe we can help each other. It may feel like the blind leading the blind, but it's all we've got!"

• *Since neither of you can claim superiority, you may be able to brainstorm solutions to common problems with your child.* Perhaps you notice that you can't have a discussion with your 13-year-old daughter without emotions escalating quickly on both sides. Maybe you can put your heads together to come up with ways you can help each other talk about emotionally charged topics without either of you losing control.

• *Before you throw up your arms in exasperation over something your child does, remind yourself that you grew up with the same challenges and yet somehow made it to adulthood okay.* Tell yourself your child may work out okay, too, despite the system's glitch. Perhaps you can think of a story from your own childhood to share with your child. I remember (this is Peg talking) my mother telling me about how her brothers had to drag her back to hear her mother read the end of *Hansel and Gretel* so she would know it turned out okay in the end. As a child who struggled with emotional control myself, I found it comforting to hear how the same problem affected my mother when she was a girl.

• *Consider taking a more systematic approach to address your weak executive skill at the same time you work on the same skill in your child.* The steps you would take to do this are:

1. Identify your child's weak skills by filling out the appropriate questionnaire in Chapter 2.
2. Identify your own weak skills by completing the questionnaire in this chapter. Make sure you're honest! It will help to complete the questionnaire with the assistance of your spouse or someone who knows you well.
3. Identify two to three recurring or repeating behaviors that your child shows that are indications of an executive skill weakness that you want to work on that matches your weak area.
4. Do the same for yourself. Identify situations where your weakness in the same executive skill interferes with effective daily functioning.
5. For yourself, identify the one place where this behavior most annoys people and identify a strategy you can use to address the problem in that situation.
6. Talk to your child about his/her specific behaviors and the situations in which they occur. Explain how you have a similar problem and talk about how you intend to work on it.
7. Together, agree on a solution to the child's problem and a cueing strategy to remind your child to use the solution.
8. Watch the behavior and apply the strategy.

We recommend this process for several reasons. First, completing the questionnaires for yourself and your child confirms that there are executive skill weaknesses you share. Second, identifying situations that cause problems for both of you helps you better understand the skill and how it affects you and your child. This may make it a little easier to empathize with your child when before you may have felt only irritation. Third, designing an intervention strategy for yourself may make it easier to identify potential strategies your child can use.

Let's walk through this process using an example of a parent and child who have weak organizational skills. Ellen Scott sees how this problem in her 13-year-old daughter, Amanda, frequently creates tension in the family. Amanda loses her assignment book and then has no place to keep track of her homework. She leaves homework on her cluttered desk at home because when she's done for the evening she doesn't put everything back in her backpack to make sure it gets to school in the morning. And she can't find favorite clothes or belongings because of the mess in her bedroom. As to herself, Ellen realizes that at least once or twice a week she sets down her cell phone in a random place that makes it difficult for her to find as well as hard for her to remember that she wants to have it with her when she leaves for work in the morning. She also keeps forgetting to recharge the phone, so even when she has it with her, the battery is often too low to use.

Ellen first decides on a strategy to help her keep track of her cell phone. Her phone allows her to program it with daily reminders, so she sets a reminder that causes the phone to ring shortly after she gets home from work. This reminds her to place the phone on the recharging dock. She also sets an alarm for the morning, just before she leaves for work, that reminds her to take the phone with her.

Now she sits down with Amanda to talk about her organizational problems. She describes how she will handle her own organizational problem and asks Amanda to identify one problem situation that she wants to tackle in a similar fashion. Amanda chooses to work first on keeping track of her assignment book. She decides that every morning when she wakes up she'll place a large neon sign on her bed that says, "Is your assignment book in your backpack?" At night she'll see the sign when she turns down the covers to go to bed. At that point she'll carry the sign over to her backpack, make sure the assignment book is in the backpack, and then lay the sign on top of the backpack so she'll remember to put it back on her bed before leaving for school in the morning.

When Overload Widens the Gap

We all know that when we're under stress our ability to cope deteriorates. The most obvious example: if you have a "short fuse" (weak emotional control) under the best of circumstances, you know you're likely to erupt more quickly and more intensely on a day like this: You were up in the middle of the night tending to your sick preschooler, then your second-grade daughter threw a fit right as the school bus was arriving at the door because she lost the toy she'd been planning to take to show-and-tell for a week, and you'd barely finished dealing with that crisis when your spouse announced his car was due for a service appointment and he needed you to drop him off at work on your way to your office. When you got to work, your boss told you that a client would be making an unexpected visit to the office to find out the status of his account and you knew you were behind schedule. If you were able to contain your emotions with your boss, your poor secretary might end up suffering the brunt of your frustrations.

Through years of working with executive skill strengths and weaknesses, we've found that in situations of stress or overload your ability to call on your executive skills may decline in general, but those skills that are most susceptible to impairment are those that were weakest to start with. We sometimes call this the "weak organ theory" (in any illness, organs that are weakest to start with are most susceptible to further breakdown). Dick has learned, for instance, to recognize that I'm under particular stress (this is Peg again) when he asks me an innocuous question and I answer him between clenched teeth. Emotional control is not my strong point. And I know when I walk into his office and find his conference table piled high with papers, folders, and books that Dick has probably overcommitted himself and his organizational skills are breaking down still further.

When your weakest executive skills seem to suffer a setback, this is a good clue that your stress level is rising. Knowing this about yourself, you may be able to put systems in place to reduce the stress or to cope with your decline in executive functioning. This could mean asking a spouse, friend, or even your child to help out in ways they might not normally, or it could mean putting goals or projects on hold while you deal with the stressful situation. Postponed projects may very well include the work you're doing with your child to improve his executive skills. Periods when you're coping with an illness in the family, financial setbacks, or marital conflicts may not be the best time to try to teach your child to clean up his bedroom. Behavior change—yours or your child's—is hard work and is most likely to be successful when undertaken in periods of calm.

Even when you're not having to manage major stressors, you should be attuned to daily situations that might impact your ability to follow through effectively with any plan you've come up with to help your child improve executive functioning. A stressful day at the office, not getting enough sleep last night, or having to fast in preparation for a medical procedure the following day can shorten your fuse or increase your impatience with your child. When these events occur, you may be able to prepare yourself by recognizing that it will take extra work on your part to remain cool, stay the course, or follow through with consequences. This will be particularly important in situations where consistency is essential. If you're working with your child to be able to take no for an answer, it's better for you to make the extra effort to hold the line than to give in and decide to try again tomorrow.

Sometimes, though, it may make sense to set aside the plan briefly. If you and your daughter have made a pact that today is the day you and she were going to plan out her science project, you may make the decision that, due to unforeseen circumstances, it's not a good day to do this. You may present the issue as having two possible solutions: "Susie, I'm feeling a little under the weather, and I know I promised to help you with your science project, but I don't think I can today. Would you like to work on it a little by yourself and go till you get stuck, or would you rather wait until tomorrow, when I'll be able to give you more help?" Sometimes these unforeseen circumstances lead children to rise to the occasion in ways that parents might not anticipate.

It's not just your stress level that can affect an intervention; it's also the stress your child may be feeling. What are some events that are likely to cause your child to feel stressed? In general, they're probably the same things that cause you to feel stressed—having too much to do with too little time to do it, being expected to do something he doesn't feel capable of doing, feeling that he is being criticized unfairly (particularly if it's for something over which he feels he has no control), or having relationship problems in general. In a child's life, this might mean having homework piled on by several teachers or being given an open-ended homework assignment that requires "thinking outside the box." Or maybe your son comes home and reports that his science teacher accused him of copying off another child's test and wouldn't listen to his explanation. Or your daughter tells you that she overheard kids talking about her in the girls' bathroom and laughing at her for being so flat chested in the eighth grade.

Any of these events can interfere with performance. Just *how* they may interfere with performance depends in part on what the child's profile of executive skill strengths and weaknesses are. The way you help your child cope may vary depending on the child's executive skills profile, although in general we recommend you acknowledge how the problem makes your child feel (what psychologists call *reflective listening*—"You must be feeling overwhelmed by the homework load," or "It must make you feel kind of powerless when you see that a teacher is not listening to your side of the story").

The good news is that if you recognize the problems for what they are—system overloads that particularly tax skills that are weak to begin with, you can intervene either before, during, or after the problem arises to minimize the fallout.

Being aware of stressors that overload the system and widen the executive skill gap is one important way to start paying attention to the fit between your child and the environment when you're trying to help your child build or enhance executive skills. Parents and teachers alter the environment to ensure a good fit all the time so that kids have the best possible chance to build competence. Modifying the environment when the task before your child taps directly into his executive skill weaknesses is particularly important. Sometimes your child can opt out of a task that is just a terrible fit for his executive skills. Other times you have to find a way to manipulate the environment, including aspects of the task itself, to make the task a good fit for your son or daughter. The next chapter will show you how.

4

···

Matching the Child to the Task

Carmen is a shy 10-year-old who has trouble thinking on her feet and feels awkward in social situations. Her Girl Scout troop is putting on a party at a local nursing home, and the scout leader has assigned troop members different roles and responsibilities for the event. They are planning on having a raffle, and she asks Carmen to collect the raffle tickets from all the nursing home residents and then to announce the numbers as they are chosen. Carmen accepts the job without saying anything, but when her mother picks her up after the meeting, she notices that her daughter is unusually quiet on the drive home. When she asks if anything is wrong, Carmen says everything is fine, but her mood remains serious throughout the evening. Finally, during the quiet time she and her mother share before bedtime, Carmen tells her about the party assignment and confesses that she really doesn't want to do what she's been asked. Her mother knows from past experience that this kind of situation can lead to stomachaches and difficulty sleeping. She suggests that she and Carmen try to think of something else she could do instead. Carmen is a very good piano player and has been practicing Christmas carols a lot lately, so her mother suggests she play the piano in the background during the party. Carmen likes this idea, knowing that enough practice will give her confidence that she can do this well. The next day her mother calls the troop leader and explains how small talk and speaking in front of a group makes Carmen nervous. She suggests that Carmen play the piano instead. Her troop leader, unaware that Carmen has this talent, accepts enthusiastically.

In the last chapter we gave you an opportunity to figure out how the fit between your executive skills and your child's can affect your interactions. You probably now have an idea of whether routine tasks that your child needs to do are even harder (for both of you) because you're strong where your child is weak or because they demand skills where you're both a bit challenged. This knowledge has a lot of power to reset the stage for better cooperation between you. It can open your eyes to approaches you hadn't considered and definitely reduces conflict. You learn to capitalize on your respective strengths and end up boosting your child's chances to develop and practice executive skills he needs.

You can see the benefits in this story of Carmen and her mother. Carmen's mom is outgoing by nature and hasn't always had a lot of patience with her daughter's reticence. But now that she understands her daughter may lack flexibility and emotional control, she quickly proposes an alternative that plays to her daughter's strengths, instead of wasting time trying to cajole her daughter to do something that Carmen would find so difficult that nothing positive could likely come from the experience.

Carmen's mother has recognized a lack of goodness of fit between her daughter and the task she was asked to do. When there is a good match between a child's executive skills and the tasks she is asked to perform, she will approach the tasks with confidence and complete them with ease. When there is not a good match, the child's response is not as predictable. Open-ended social situations are anxiety provoking for Carmen, and her anticipation of them causes unpleasant physical symptoms. Fortunately for Carmen, Girl Scouts is a leisure activity and therefore more flexible than some of the other settings in which kids have to perform, such as the classroom. Carmen's mother could try to alter or replace the task that her daughter was expected to do in order to improve the fit between child and task.

Of course another option would have been for Carmen to opt out of this event altogether. This is always one alternative with discretionary activities. The challenge is always to weigh the pros and cons: you don't want your child to feel like she fails at everything she tries; on the other hand, you don't want to deny her the opportunities for growth that almost any activity offers a developing child. So if you can find a way for her to participate and still feel competent, she will likely come out of the experience with new and/or improved skills of some type or another.

Parents often labor under the misconception that children develop self-esteem when we praise them for attributes like being smart or gifted or athletic. Praise can be helpful (although there are rules for effective praise that will be discussed in Chapter 8). In fact, a primary way children develop self-esteem is by tackling obstacles and overcoming them. The more arenas they test their skills in, the more confident they become that they can handle new obstacles when they arise. The art of parenting involves being able to identify with some degree of accuracy which challenges are at just the right level for a child to be able to succeed with a little effort.

Sometimes it may be obvious that the best choice is to steer your child away from a particular situation altogether, such as when the entire setting demands a number of executive skills he doesn't have. That's why many churches have children come for the beginning of a church service and go off to Sunday school before their attention and impulse control are taxed too much. Wise parents gauge family gatherings based on what they know their children can tolerate, finding babysitters for events such as weddings when the probability is great that their children will disrupt the ceremony. Where there is not a good match between the demands of a task and normative behavior for a particular age, adults take steps to provide alternative experiences. This may become a little more difficult to handle if your child is delayed compared to his age group. As a parent, it's your job to step in and make decisions that protect your child. Here's an example:

Sherry, age 8, has been invited to her first sleepover, part of her friend Laura's birthday party. Her mother knows that her daughter has a hard time falling asleep, needs to sleep with the light on, and worries about sounds she hears in the night. Often she wakes up in the middle of the night and comes into her parents' room just to make sure they're there. She and Sherry's dad have been working on this with her, and they've seen improvement, but they don't think she's ready for a sleepover in a strange home yet. Her mom calls Laura's mom and explains the situation, and then she tells Sherry that she will let her go to the party but that she'll need to come home at bedtime since there is a family event the next day that they want her to participate in. Sherry had been looking forward to the party, but her mother can tell she's relieved when she finds she won't be spending the night.

Unfortunately, not all tasks or situations your child faces during the day will be amenable to modifications to suit his existing executive skills. School is certainly an example.

> Roger, another 10-year-old, hates to write. His handwriting is poor, the mechanical act of writing is slow and laborious for him, and he can never think of anything to write about. The last problem is the worst! He sits and stares at the blank sheet of paper in front of him and feels helpless. The frustration mounts inside him until he blows up. "I can't do this stupid homework!" he screams at his mother. "I don't know why Mrs. Carson keeps giving us writing. I'm not going to do it, and you can't make me!" He crumples the paper in front of him, throws his pencil at the wall, and storms off to his bedroom to play video games. His mother throws up her arms in her own frustration. *Why does Roger act this way?* she wonders. When she described his behavior to his teacher, she was genuinely surprised. At school, Roger never said "boo" (although the teacher did admit he often lingered over writing assignments to the point where she had to send them home with him for homework).

Roger, too, has trouble with flexibility and emotional control (along with weak metacognitive skills, which means he has trouble figuring out a reasonable solution to the problem in front of him), and the task he's been asked to do taps into all his executive skill weaknesses. Because this is schoolwork and his executive skill weaknesses make it hard for him to master an important academic skill, however, Roger's mother can't just try to find something else for Roger to do in the same situation, as Carmen's mother did. In Roger's case, it will be necessary to find ways to alter the writing task to make it more manageable for him. The good news is that there are usually a lot more ways to do this than may be immediately evident:

- Roger's mother could talk with him about the topic before he starts writing to help him generate ideas and organize his thoughts.
- She could have him dictate his work to remove the manual labor that makes writing that much harder for him.
- Or maybe the teacher would be willing to reduce the task—for example, by requiring him to write two sentences rather than a complete paragraph, or one paragraph rather than three.

These are just a few of the possibilities. A lot more may suggest themselves to Roger's mother and his teacher once they put their minds to solving the problem. But if the solutions they come up with are to be truly effective, they have to know exactly what they're dealing with, which means pulling apart the task, the environment in which it has to be done, and the child's abilities:

1. *When you know your child has executive skill weaknesses, pay close attention to the child's emotional and behavioral responses to tasks assigned.* Carmen couldn't speak up to her troop leader and tell her she didn't want to do the job she'd been assigned. She didn't even want to tell her mother at first, but in the quiet of her bedtime during a nightly ritual when she was used to sharing her deepest thoughts with her mother, she was able to make her confession. And Roger, too, acted very different at home than at school. At school, surrounded by his classmates, he would have been embarrassed to throw the kind of tantrum he routinely exhibited at home. If Carmen's mom hadn't been paying attention to the slight but perceptible shift in her behavior on the way home from the Girl Scout meeting, she might have missed the fact that something was wrong and never figured out that Carmen had been asked to do something she found very difficult to do. Carmen might have ended up being set up for failure, which would have exposed her to the potential damage discussed earlier. If Roger's mother had just assumed her son was being rebellious and trying to get out of homework, she may never have known how hard writing tasks felt to him, because the teacher hadn't noticed a problem at school. The longer the problem remained unaddressed, the harder writing might have become for Roger and the more dedicated he might have become to avoiding situations that required writing.

2. *When your child seems to be avoiding a task, consider the possibility that the child can't do it.* Children react to challenging tasks with a wide variety of different emotional responses and behaviors that might not immediately signal that they *can't* do what they've been asked to do. Carmen tended to withdraw and develop stomachaches. Roger acted out. Other kids are masters at work avoidance. They get up to sharpen their pencils, dawdle over the pencil sharpener, and find any excuse to do something other than write if writing is hard for them. Or they may attempt to

engage a classmate, sibling, teacher, or parent in conversation or allow themselves to become distracted by anything going on in their immediate environment. They may become silly or defiant or complain of fatigue (in fact, effortful tasks do have the effect of inducing fatigue in some children). Kids do all these things in lieu of saying "I don't know how to do this."

Of course, some children do just this—say they don't know how to do the task—but all too often the response from parents or teachers to that direct statement of truth is "Of *course* you know how to do this. This is *easy*." This, unfortunately, has the effect of making the child feel that much "dumber" because he's just been told that the task he doesn't know how to do is, in fact, easy. If you've said this to your child regarding certain tasks, ask yourself whether these are tasks that involve executive skills in which you are strong while your child is weak. If so, the temptation to say it is your cue to look more closely at the task itself and why your child can't handle it. It's the job of adults (parents and teachers particularly) to identify what about the task led to the emotional or behavioral response so that they can understand the behavior in front of them and the nature of the obstacles that led to the behavior.

3. *Figure out what executive skills the task requires and ask yourself whether your child possesses these skills.* Of course, you don't need to do this for every chore or homework assignment your child has to do, but if your child is resisting a particular chore or activity, it makes sense to consider whether part of this resistance comes from the poor match between the task and your child's skills. Since you determined what your child's executive skill weaknesses are when you completed the rating scale in Chapter 2, you may be able simply to ask yourself whether the task your child is balking at requires any of those weak skills. Alternatively, you could start with the task and go down the list of executive skills to determine which ones play a prominent role in the task at hand.

Let's take room cleaning as an example. This is a task that almost all parents expect their children to be able to accomplish, but if you look at the executive skills required, you can see that there are any number of ways a child with weak executive skills might get tripped up. For children to be completely independent with respect to room cleaning, at a minimum, the following executive skills are required:

- Task initiation—the child has to be able to start the task without reminders.
- Sustained attention—the child has to be able to stick with the task long enough to get it done.
- Planning/prioritization—the child has to have a plan of attack and a way to make decisions about what's important and what's not important (for example, what needs to be saved and what should be thrown out).
- Organization—the child has to have some way of managing his belongings so that everything has a place.

When a task requires multiple executive skills, you may be able to determine that the breakdown occurs when the child has to use a weak skill. You can then build in supports to work around the weak skill. If task initiation is the problem, then you and your child agree on when the room will be cleaned and what kind of reminder your child would like to get started. If sustained attention is the problem, then you and your child could break room cleaning into pieces and have a plan for when each piece will be done. If planning is the problem, then you and your child could sit down and make a list of the steps involved in room cleaning and turn it into a checklist. And if organization is the problem, then you might look at how to help your child design her bedroom to make it easier for her to organize her belongings. These examples are exactly the types of things you'll learn to do in Part III of this book.

4. *Figure out whether something in the environment is making the task difficult for your child.* For youngsters with weak executive skills or with skills that are just emerging, fairly minor things in the environment can disrupt their ability to use those skills. Distractions, such as the television being on in the background or an interesting conversation to eavesdrop on, can be an interference. For some children, being observed while they perform a difficult task can be enough to stop them in their tracks—especially if they feel they are being judged. If you're having trouble getting your child to practice the piano, then refraining from offering "constructive advice" while the child is practicing is probably a good idea.

On the other hand, in some cases leaving children completely on their own to perform a task can impede the process. Children with weak sustained attention, for example, are susceptible to distractions (internal and external) that draw them off-task. For children with weak planning skills or inflexible children, being left on their own may leave them not knowing how to start the task or how to progress through it. This is particularly a problem when the task is open-ended (that is, where there are multiple possible routes or multiple possible solutions). For many children, being left on their own to complete a task makes the task appear overwhelming to them—it has too many steps or they think it will take them too long to complete it, and without someone cheering them on or offering encouragement or positive feedback, they quickly become discouraged and give up.

You may also be perplexed by your child's ability to use a particular executive skill effectively in one situation but fail to use it in other situations. Sometimes the amount of structure a situation imposes makes the difference. For instance, a child may be able to do a writing assignment in school (where he is surrounded by other children writing and knows the teacher is keeping an eye on him and can check in with him periodically to see how he's doing or offer small suggestions) but may not be able to do a similar writing assignment at home (where there is less supervision and he is less confident that his mom or dad will be able to help him when he gets stuck). If you can identify what factors contribute to success in one situation or failure in another, you may be able to "tweak the environment" to enhance the likelihood of success.

A significant factor affecting a child's ability to use executive skills well is the child's degree of interest in the task at hand or the child's motivation to achieve suc-cess. Kids who routinely forget to take homework assignments to school have no trouble remembering to take in a CD they want to share with a friend. Kids who for-get to stay after school to get help from their math teacher to study for a test have no trouble remembering that this is the day a parent said they could go to the mall after school to use their gift certificate. If this sounds like your child, it doesn't necessarily mean that he or she doesn't have weak working memory—it just means that the extra motivation the child has to engage in a particular activity overrides the child's naturally weak memory. Knowing that children can use executive skills more effec-tively when the motivation is sufficient, you may be able to find ways to link task performance to motivating factors that entice your child to make the increased effort necessary to accomplish tasks that require them to use executive skills that don't come easily to them.

Chapter 6 will describe in much greater detail environmental factors that can prevent children from using executive skills, as well as offer suggestions for how to modify the environment to help children be more successful. Chapter 8 will talk more about how to motivate children to use and grow weak executive skills.

5. *If your child can do the task sometimes but not all the time, this may simply mean that you've identified an executive skill weakness.* There is a big difference between being able to do a task and being able to do that task *consistently.* Those of you who are organizationally challenged may understand this quite well if we explain this in the context of keeping your desk neat and tidy. Sure, you're perfectly capable of cleaning off your desk. You *know how* to do this. For instance, you may decide what items you want to keep on your desk and then take everything else, one piece at a time, and decide what to do with it (throw it out, file it, put it in the to-do box, give it to someone else to handle, etc.). Once you've cleaned your desk, however, think about how hard it is, day in and day out, to *keep it clean.* This is what kids are often up against as they encounter tasks that tap their executive skill weaknesses: they may know what to do or how to do it, but to do it consistently, day in and day out, as long as their parents or teachers require them to do it is a whole other story!

If you encounter situations like this with your child, you have a few options. You can try to stay on top of a situation so that it doesn't get out of hand. For a child with organizational problems, for instance, this may mean spending 10 minutes at the end of every day picking up the playroom rather than waiting until the weekend and tackling a bigger mess. For a child with time management problems, this may mean imposing a schedule on him for the project that he thinks he can finish in 30 minutes when you know it's going to take several hours.

In some cases, though, you may find it best to "pick your battles." This may mean letting things slide at times—for example, skipping the room cleaning on a night when your child was stressed out by homework or had an extra long sports practice. Children who have problems with emotional control are particularly sus-ceptible to stress from a variety of sources that affects not only their ability to control their emotions but also their ability to use other executive skills. Fatigue, hunger, overstimulation, a bad day at school, an unexpected change in plans all can impact their ability to mobilize resources and executive skills and may require on-the-fly adjustment by parents in helping them manage their behavior. If parents find themselves letting things slide too frequently, though, they may need to look at whether they can reduce the "triggers" that set their children off. Whenever possible, it's probably preferable to reduce demands rather than let kids off the hook altogether. Instead of having them spend 10 minutes tidying up the playroom, for instance, this might mean having them just pick up the Legos and leave the other toys until tomorrow.

6. *If your child has handled the task some of the time, figure out what made success possible.* Maybe you've heard yourself say something like "You complained about this the last time you had to do this and you eventually were able to do it, so stop complaining and get to work." If you've said this, you may be overlooking some important factors. First of all, how much and what kind of support did you offer the last time that enabled your child to complete the task successfully? You may have done any number of things to make the task easier for the child without even realizing you were doing so:

- Did you talk with your child about what he had to do before he got started (what we sometimes call "priming the pump")?
- Did you break the task down for your child?
- Did you give your child permission to work for just 5 minutes before taking a break?

These are just a few of the possibilities. If you feel confounded by your child's inconsistent ability to accomplish a certain task, try to review the successful experiences and the failures. You might even jot down various environmental factors involved in each in two columns and then compare to see where the keys to success might lie.

7. *If the child seems to have the executive skills to do the task, is the problem that the child doesn't believe he can succeed?* There is one other important variable that helps determine goodness of fit. This is the child's own estimation of his ability to succeed. If you've examined the task closely, and then compared the skills the task requires with your child's skills, and also looked at the environment in which the task has to be done, and you still can't figure out why your child shouldn't be able to do the job at hand, it may be simply a lack of confidence on the part of the child. Children can lack confidence for a number of reasons:

- The task looks too big and they can't see beyond the size of the task to see that each individual step the task requires is within their ability to perform.
- They have tried and failed at so many other things that they lump this task in with those and assume they will fail at this too.

- Their efforts have been met with criticism in the past and they don't want to risk this happening again—this is particularly true with children with perfectionist tendencies (who often have parents with perfectionist tendencies), since no matter how well they perform a task, it never quite meets either their expectations or those of others they want to please or impress.
- Someone has always jumped in and rescued them as soon as they encounter an obstacle, so they've never learned that they can overcome obstacles on their own (or with minimal assistance).

Sometimes a task is well within a child's range of competence and you see this clearly. But if your child doesn't believe she's capable of performing the task, she's likely to engage in the same set of diversions that she would use when confronted with a task she genuinely is unable to perform. Fortunately, you can handle these two kinds of situations in the same way—alter the task in some small way to help the child experience quick success. When the task is truly within the child's repertoire, success usually comes more quickly and the problem abates more rapidly, as long as the child sees her success and gets positive feedback about that success from others.

In many cases, the way to handle these situations is to help your child get started on the task, whatever it is, and let him know *you won't let him fail* (that is, you'll offer support as needed as he progresses through the task). You may find it helpful to use the analogy of learning to ride a bike after the training wheels are removed. Let your child know you'll help him in the same way you held onto the back of the bike to steady him until he told you it was OK to let go. If the task truly is within your child's repertoire, then that assurance plus the early support should be sufficient and your child will quickly let you know "it's OK to let go." This approach can be particularly useful when children have homework they don't think they can do. Get them started, give them small hints and quiet words of encouragement, and praise them for sticking with it or trying hard. And jump in with more substantive support if they start getting discouraged or hit a roadblock.

Offering to practice or rehearse the problem situation is another way to help your child gain confidence. Maybe your son wants to call and invite a friend over but he's not sure how to do this. Give him a script and then role-play the situation with him until he feels comfortable making the call. You may want to practice with several possible outcomes (for example, how to handle it when the friend turns down the invitation for different reasons), so that your child is prepared for a number of alternative endings.

Whatever the details may be, when there's a poor fit between the task or the environment and the child's executive skill profile, children will try to take control of the situation, either by escaping or avoiding it. In the scenarios described earlier, Carmen and Roger responded by trying to avoid the situation. A child with Asperger syndrome who is inflexible and has trouble handling casual conversations reshapes the situation to match his skills by dominating the conversation with talk of his own interests. Even kids without Asperger syndrome* who are inflexible sometimes have this problem and handle it in the same way. Children who have weak emotional control or poor impulse control often have difficulty handling situations in which there is a lot happening around them or when events unfold quickly. They may handle these situations by walking out or retreating to a quiet corner. My youngest son (this is Peg talking) as a preschooler used to start misbehaving when friends came over and stayed too long. He didn't know how to tell them to go home, but he knew that I would read his behavioral cues and tell his friends that the play date was over. In Part II of the book, we will lay out a set of conditions that you need to understand to make adjustments to improve the fit between your child and the tasks your child is asked to do.

---

*While "Asperger's disorder" is the preferred terminology of the American Psychiatric Association in DSM-IV-TR, the condition is most commonly known as "Asperger syndrome," so we will use that term here.

Part II

LAYING A FOUNDATION
THAT CAN HELP

5

Ten Principles for Improving Your Child's Executive Skills

By now you should have a pretty good idea of how important executive skills are to a child's ability to meet the demands typically placed on kids of his or her age. You're probably forming a clearer picture of where your child's strengths and weaknesses lie and why your child has trouble with certain tasks but glides through others with ease. You may already be coming up with ideas for how to capitalize on those strengths so that your child acts as smart as you know your son or daughter is—and a lot less scattered. And we'd bet the level of conflict is already a little lower now that you know how to maximize the fit between you and your child and how to get around the inevitable divides.

In this chapter we've distilled all this background into 10 principles that should guide you in helping your child grow and develop. You can use them to apply the strategies in Part III to your child's unique circumstances and characteristics or to design your own strategies. Either way, they are the "rules" for helping a child manage tasks that are currently challenging, for developing executive skills in which the child is lagging, and for encouraging your child to practice executive skills to maximize his potential in these areas. You'll read more about the most important of these principles in the rest of Part II.

1. *Teach* deficient skills rather than expecting the child to acquire them through observation or osmosis.

It does appear that some children have a natural capacity for using executive skills effectively, while others stumble and struggle if left on their own. This may not be all that different from other skills, such as learning how to read. A small percentage of children seem to teach themselves how to read, while the vast majority require exposure to formal instruction. Another small percentage of kids don't seem to acquire the skill quickly or smoothly, even with classroom instruction in reading. Many parents and teachers foster executive skill development through what psychologists call *incidental learning*—that is, they provide loose structures, models, and occasional prompts and cues, and that's all that's needed. Or maybe that was all that was needed in simpler times, when the demands on children were less and where the amount of supervision and support teachers and parents could provide was greater.

In this day and age, however, most children struggle at one point or another with some task that requires a level of executive functioning that's beyond them. To respond to this more complex world, we can't leave executive skill development to chance. We need to provide our kids with direct instruction—defining problem behaviors, identifying goal behaviors, and then developing and implementing an instructional sequence that includes close supervision at first, followed by a gradual fading of prompts and supports. We'll describe this process, which is aimed at tackling specific tasks, in more detail in Chapter 7. But there are other, more natural ways to teach executive skills, through scaffolding and even games you can play that encourage the development of executive skills overall rather than by targeting a specific task that requires certain skills. This approach is also described more fully in Chapter 7. Also note how this principle relates to principle number 3. When you teach skills by modifying the task to make it manageable, you're starting with the external, but the goal is to end up with internalization of the skill taught in that task so that the child has it in his repertoire and can apply it freely on his own to other tasks requiring it in the future.

2. Consider your child's developmental level.

We don't expect 5-year-olds to plan and prepare the lunches they take to daycare, we don't expect 10-year-olds to pack for summer camp on their own, and we don't expect 14-year-olds to live in their own apartment. Yet in our clinical practice we see a lot of parents who hold unrealistic expectations for their child's level of independence. We once worked with a parent, for instance, who expected her 8-year-old daughter to remember all on her own to take her asthma medication each morning, something most children need help remembering at least through the upper elementary grades, if not longer. And we routinely work with parents of high school freshmen who are irritated because their children do not have a clear plan for the college they want to go to after they graduate and understand what they need to do to get into that college. It is not unusual, in our experience, for even high school seniors to need assistance with this process from parents, guidance counselors, or both.

Understanding what's normal at any given age so that you don't expect too much from your child is the first step in addressing executive skill weaknesses. We included a table in Chapter 2 (p. 30) that lists the typical ages at which we expect children to perform tasks that involve executive skills. We have also included more detailed checklists in Part III that you can use to identify where your child stands in terms of developing specific executive skills.

But knowing what's typical for any given age is only part of the process. When your child's skills are delayed or deficient based on age, you'll need to step in and intervene at whatever level your child is functioning at now. While a normal 12-year-old may be able to pick up his room by himself with a weekly schedule and a reminder or two (or three!), if your 12-year-old has never picked up his room by himself in his life, then the structures and strategies that work with most 12-year-olds will probably not work with yours. You will need to match the task demands to the child's actual developmental level if that's different from his peers or from what you would like it to be. The same table in Chapter 2 should help you get an idea of the developmental age of your child, at least as far as the particular executive skills you're worried about are concerned.

3. Move from the external to the internal.

As we've mentioned, you acted largely as your child's frontal lobes when your child was really small. All executive skills training begins with something *outside* the child. Before you taught your child not to run into the road, you stayed with him and held his hand when the two of you reached a street corner to make sure that didn't happen. Eventually, because you repeated the rule *Look both ways before crossing*, your child internalized the rule, then you observed your child following the rule, and now your son can handle crossing the street by himself. In all kinds of ways, you organize and structure your child's environment to compensate for the executive skills your child has not yet developed. When you decide to help your child develop more effective executive skills, therefore, you should always begin by changing things outside the child before moving on to strategies that require the child to change. Some examples:

- Cueing a child to brush her teeth before she goes to bed rather than expecting her to remember to do this on her own.
- Keeping tasks very brief rather than expecting a young child to work for a long time to complete a chore.
- Keeping birthday parties small to avoid overstimulating a child who struggles with emotional control.
- Making a toddler or preschooler hold your hand when walking through a busy parking lot.

4. Remember that the external includes changes you can make in the environment, the task, or the way you interact with your child.

Be sure you consider all three possibilities whenever you're going to try to modify something external to the child to make a task manageable and encourage the development of executive skills. You can make minor changes in the physical or social environment. This can be something as simple as having a child with ADHD do her homework in the kitchen, where she can be monitored and given reminders and encouragement to stay on track. For a child with weak emotional control, it might mean finding younger playmates or limiting play dates to one child at a time or having a parent or babysitter on hand to supervise beyond the age when this is typically done for kids. You can also alter the task in numerous ways so that the end result is achieved but the route is different from the one that's gotten you nowhere so far; that's what much of Part III of this book shows you how to do. Finally, you can change the way you (or other adults, like teachers) interact with your child. You may already be doing some of the last now that you know how your executive skills compare to your child's, but there are more specific ideas for interacting differently, as well as modifying the environment or the task, in Chapter 6.

5. Use rather than fight the child's innate drive for mastery and control.

As any parent of a 2-year-old knows, from a very early age children work hard to control their own lives. They do this by achieving mastery and by working to get what they want when they want it. The mastery part is a delight for parents to watch: the persistence with which an infant practices pulling herself to a stand or climbing stairs is replaced just a few years down the road by learning to ride a two-wheeled bike and several years later by learning to drive a car. Parents tend to be a little more ambivalent about the ways their children work to get what they want when they want it, because what *they* want is sometimes in conflict with what parents want.

Nonetheless, there are ways you can support your child's agenda while remaining in charge. These include:

- Creating routines and schedules so that your child knows what will happen when and will accept them as a part of his everyday life. This is particularly important for activities that occur daily, such as mealtimes, bedtimes, chores, and homework. This carves out certain times of the day or certain activities where the child understands that the parents' agenda holds sway. When you preempt that "space," your child is less likely to stake a claim to it and will therefore be less resistant to following the plan you've designed.
- Building in choices, to give your child some control. This might include a choice of what chores the child will do, when the child will do them, or in what order.
- Practicing difficult tasks in small steps and increasing the demand only gradually.

- Using negotiation. The goal here is to move away from the "automatic no," while ensuring that the child has to pass through a "have to" to get to the "want to." This have-to-to-want-to progression is also known as "Grandma's law," because grandmothers have always been adept at getting children to complete a chore before the kids are allowed to have one of their delicious home-baked chocolate chip cookies.

6. Modify tasks to match your child's capacity to exert effort.

Some tasks require more effort than others. This is as true for adults as it is for children. Think of that task at your office that you keep putting off—you know, the one that you can think of a million things you have to do that are more pressing than that one. Or think of that chore you've been hounding your spouse about for weeks. It's not that he or she—or you, for that matter—*can't* do it.

In fact, though, there are two kinds of effortful tasks: ones that you're not very good at and ones that you are very capable of doing but you just don't like doing. The same is true for children, and different strategies apply depending on which kind of task is under consideration.

If we're talking about tasks the child is not very good at, you handle them by breaking them down into small steps and starting with either the first step and proceeding forward or the last step and proceeding backward, and you don't proceed to the next step until the child has mastered the previous step. Take bed-making as an example. Beginning at the end would mean doing the entire task except the last step (putting the pillows on the bed after having put the bedspread in place). Starting at the beginning might mean asking the child simply to straighten the top sheet. You praise the child for doing a good job and restrict the child's responsibility to that first step until that step becomes second nature or so easy the child can do it with her eyes closed, and then you move on to the next step.

But really, it's the second kind of effortful task that parents tend to have strong feelings about. These are the ones where you might accuse your children of "just deciding they don't like them." Our feeling is that if the task has become a battleground between you and your child, it's probably gone beyond a simple decision on the part of the child that the task is distasteful. Our advice is: if you've fought that battle a couple of times and didn't win, it's best to change the nature of the battle. The goal is then to teach your child to exert effort by getting him to override the desire to quit or do anything else that's preferable. The way to do this is to make the first step *easy enough* so that it doesn't feel particularly hard to the child and to immediately follow that first step with a reward. The reward is there to ensure that there's a payoff for the child for expending the small amount of effort it takes to complete the first step. You then gradually increase the amount of effort the child has to expend to achieve the reward. This is done either by increasing the task demands or by increasing the amount of time you expect the child to work before the reward can be earned.

When we work with parents of children who resist tasks that take effort, we've found it helpful to have them use a scale, say, from 1 to 10, when gauging how hard the task feels to the child. Ten on this scale is a task the child can do but that feels *very, very hard*, while 1 on this scale is something that requires *virtually no effort at all*. The goal is to design or modify the task so it feels like a 3.

As an example, cleaning my study (this is Peg talking now) feels like climbing Mt. McKinley to me (and I'm not a mountain climber), in part because it feels like it will take forever. Cleaning the entire study, then, is a 10 on my effort scale. Could I spend one minute working on getting it clean? Sure, that would be a breeze—so that would be a 1 on the scale. What would be a 3? Oh, maybe working for 10 or 15 minutes. Sure, it'll take me longer to clean my study than if I could do the whole job at once, but it'll get done faster than if I never tackled the job at all!

In a similar way, you can help your child use this scale to plot how to do the work that needs to get done. Let's say the one job you expect your 13-year-old son to do steadily throughout the summer is mow the lawn. And let's say you find yourself hounding him week after week to get it done. You finally realize that he avoids it because he finds it incredibly boring (and therefore requiring a lot of effort). You may find it helpful to explain the 10-point scale to him, ask him to rate lawn mowing, and then ask him what could be done to lower lawn mowing from a 10 to a 3. His first answer might be "Get me a sit-down mower with cool gadgets." Once you explain why this is out of the question, you might get him to identify how much time spent mowing the lawn might feel like a 3 to him or whether there's a reward he might want to work for that would help move the task down the rating scale.

This scale can also be applied to aversive homework assignments. You could get your daughter to begin homework planning by rating each assignment in terms of how hard she thinks it is. Then she could decide on the order in which she wants to do the assignments based on their rating—and you might encourage her to build in small breaks for the ones with higher ratings (or even switch off between easy and difficult tasks).

7. Use incentives to augment instruction.

Incentives are rewards, plain and simple. They can be as simple as a word of praise or as elaborate as a point system that enables a child to earn rewards on a daily, weekly, or monthly basis.

For some tasks—and some children—mastery of the task is incentive enough. Most children naturally want to master things like learning to pull themselves to a stand or learning to climb stairs, learning to ride a bike, or learning to drive a car. Many tasks we expect children to do lack built-in incentives, although this varies somewhat from child to child. We've met children, for instance, who love to help their moms tidy up the house or their dads clean the garage. The reward comes either from the chance to spend time with a parent, the chance to do "grown-up things," or, less commonly, the satisfaction that comes from seeing the final product (such as a clean house or garage). For many other children, the same tasks are so aversive that they go to great lengths to avoid them. Homework is another example. It's the rare child who can't wait to get home and get started on homework, but for some the grade they will earn on homework well done—or the humiliation they will avoid from getting a low grade—is sufficient to propel them to do homework assignments promptly and well. For many of the children we work with, however, the rewards and punishments associated with homework are not enough to make them willing to do it without putting up a fight first. If you have a child like this, you may want to think about additional incentives you could use to get your child through homework without its becoming a major battleground.

Incentives have the effect of making the effort of learning a skill and the effort of performing a task less aversive. We will talk about this more in Chapter 8, but rewards have an energizing effect on behavior. They give us something to look forward to that motivates us to persist with difficult tasks and that helps us combat any negative thoughts or feelings we have about the task at hand. I have fond memories (this is Peg talking) of the homemade ice cream my father used to make as a special treat on hot summer days in my childhood. Taking my turn along with my brothers at the hand crank (despite having weak arm muscles!) was well worth it, knowing the reward that awaited me at the end of my hard work.

Finally, placing an incentive after the task teaches the child to delay gratification—a valuable skill in its own right. Chapter 8 will describe a process for creating incentive systems to accompany skill instruction.

8. Provide just enough support for the child to be successful.

This appears to be so simple as to be self-evident, but in fact the implementation of this principle may be trickier than it appears. The principle includes two components that are of equal weight—(1) *just enough support* and (2) *for the child to be successful*. Parents and other adults who work with children tend to make two kinds of mistakes. They either provide too much support, which means the child is successful but fails to develop the ability to perform the task independently, or they provide too little support, so the child fails—and, again, never develops the ability to perform the task independently.

Here's a simple example. When children are ready to learn to open doors by themselves, we stop doing it for them but stand by ready to intervene at the first point where the child stops succeeding. Maybe the child can put his hand on the doorknob but doesn't know how to turn it. You, his mother or father, then put your hand gently over his and turn his hand and the doorknob until it opens. The next time the child encounters a closed door, maybe he can begin to turn it but he can't turn the knob far enough to make it open. Again, you put your hand on his, but only after he's attempted to turn the handle unsuccessfully. Through repetitions, the child eventually can open the door on his own. If, however, you insisted on continuing to pull the door open for your child, he'd never learn to do it on his own. If you stood there and let your child's frustration mount as he tried to no avail to open the door, he'd learn nothing about opening the door—except maybe that this was an unpleasant effort to avoid at all costs.

The same principle applies with any task you want your child to master. Determine how far she can get in the task on her own and then intervene—don't do the task for her, though; just offer her enough support (physical or verbal, depending on the task) to get her over the hump and moving on to success. This may take some practice, and it certainly takes close observation, but you'll get the hang of it.

9. Keep supports and supervision in place until the child achieves mastery or success.

We see parents who know how to break down tasks, teach skills, and reinforce success, and yet their children still fail to acquire the skills they want them to gain. More often than not, this is because of a failure to apply this principle and/or the next one. These parents set up a process or a procedure, see that it's working, and then back out of the picture, expecting the child to keep succeeding independently. One of the more common examples we see is the system that parents put in place to help their children get organized. They may walk them through a process of cleaning their desk, for instance, or they may buy them the notebooks or binders they need to organize their schoolwork, and even help them decide how they will use those notebooks, but they are too quick to expect their children to maintain the organizing scheme on their own.

We've had friends tell us that the Franklin Planner people used to say it takes 3 weeks for people to learn a habit. We're not sure whether there's a research base to support this or even whether it's true for adults, but for kids—especially those with executive skill deficits—this is probably too optimistic a timeline, at least if they're hoping the executive skill will be fully operational in that time. We routinely encourage parents to be alert for small signs of progress. The more precise you are in defining the problem to begin with, the more likely you are to see that progress. Before you begin to implement any of the interventions described in this book, or even one you come up with on your own, you may want to take a few minutes to write down exactly what the problem looks like—or sounds like (as in the case of temper tantrums)—right now. Describe the behavior in precise terms (for example, *forgets to hand in homework assignments; cries whenever there's an unexpected change in plans*), and either estimate or count how often it happens or how long it lasts. If it's a behavior that involves intensity (like a temper tantrum), you can rate it on a scale from *mild* to *severe*. Periodically (that is, every few weeks), you may want to pull out what you wrote and see if the progress is visible. We provide a worksheet to help you monitor improvement at the end of this chapter.

We should point out, however, that in the very early stages of attempting to change a behavior, it can sometimes get worse before it gets better. If your child cries at bedtime unless you agree to lie down with him until he falls asleep, and you decide to try to extinguish that behavior, you will likely find that the crying increases in duration or intensity before it begins to decline. Any behavioral intervention designed to address problems with emotional control or response inhibition—particularly if your strategy involves ignoring one set of behaviors while trying to teach replacement behaviors—is particularly likely to result in an increase in the problem before improvement becomes evident.

The more carefully you design (and measure) the intervention, the sooner you are likely to see progress. In our experience some parents are better able to implement precise interventions and record-keeping than others. For those who are not so precise, using periodic "check-ups" should help you see that progress is, indeed, occurring.

10. When you do stop the supports, supervision, and incentives, fade them gradually, never abruptly.

Even if you stick with the supports you put in place long enough to allow your child to learn to do the task or use the skill independently, you may be tempted to cut them off all at once. Instead, you need to fade them so that the child can achieve gradual independence with the skill. Let's go back to the bike-riding analogy we talked about in Chapter 2. If you've ever taught a child to ride a bike, you know that you start out holding on to the back of the bike to keep it upright and every once in a while as your child practices you let go for a second or two to test whether the child can keep the bike going without too much wobbling. If so, you gradually let go for longer and longer. You don't hold on to the back constantly and then suddenly just let 'er fly and expect the child and bike to keep going without a crash.

Remember principle number 8: *Provide just enough support for the child to be successful.* Don't keep cueing or prompting your child when he doesn't need you to do that. But don't go from everything to nothing either!

We'll talk more about the fading process in the next three chapters, and in Part III you'll see the process in action in detailed illustrations.

You should be able to rely on these principles whenever you're deciding how to tackle a problem task with your child or whenever you want to hone an overall skill. In fact, you might find it helpful to review these principles anytime you find yourself stumped or stalled while using the strategies in Part III. Sometimes we forget how important it is to stick to the ground rules when life and its demands—on us and our kids—gets complicated.

Three Ways to Instill Executive Skills

Embedded in these principles is a way to view any behavior you want to change, including the acquisition and use of executive skills. Behavior management experts often call this the ABC model. A in this model stands for *antecedent*, B for *behavior*, and C for *consequences*. The idea is that there are three opportunities to take measures to elicit or change the behavior as desired: by changing what comes before it (the external factors, or environment), by aiming directly at the behavior itself (through teaching), and by imposing consequences (incentives or penalties). In Chapter 6, we'll talk about modifying the environment to reduce problems with executive skills, by focusing on the antecedents to behavior—those external conditions that make executive skill problems either better or worse. In Chapter 7 we turn to the behavior itself and show you how children can be taught directly to use executive skills. Finally, in Chapter 8, we talk about using motivators to encourage children to use executive skills. Once you've read those chapters, you'll have what you need to design your own interventions to improve your child's executive functioning—or a solid base of understanding that will help you make the most of the interventions we've created for you and present in Part III.

HOW MUCH PROGRESS ARE WE MAKING?

Date	Executive skill	Precise description of behavior (What does it look like/ sound like?)	Frequency (How often does the behavior occur?—times per day, per week, etc.)	Duration (How long does it last?)	Intensity (On a scale of 1 to 5, how intense is the behavior?)
Follow-up date		Does the behavior still look/sound the same?	How often does it happen now?	How long does it last now?	How intense is it now?
Follow-up #2					

6

Modifying the Environment

A Is for *Antecedent*

Jonas, age 4, was a challenging child from birth. He was colicky as an infant, had irregular sleep patterns, was a fussy eater, and as soon as he could communicate a preference, complained about tags on his clothing, tight-fitting pants, and the seams in his socks. His parents found he fell apart at family parties, and they could almost predict to the minute when the meltdown would come. Temper tantrums seemed to arise out of nowhere—except his parents noticed they were more likely to start when he was hungry or tired or overstimulated. They seemed to be the only way Jonas knew to manage his emotions. Gradually, his parents figured out ways to reduce the problems. As much as possible, they put him on a regular schedule—wake and sleep times, mealtimes, and baths all occurred at the same time every day. They limited his television viewing, cutting out cartoons that had any whiff of violence, and they built in bedtime rituals. Play dates were restricted to one child at a time, and they never lasted more than 1½ hours. When they were invited to family parties, they arrived a little late and left a little early—and, if necessary, one of them would take Jonas for a walk halfway through the party. As a result of these changes to their family patterns, Jonas's tantrums and meltdowns diminished dramatically.

You may be familiar enough with the individual executive skills we've described to recognize that Jonas has problems with emotional control. The methods that Jonas's parents put in place to help reduce his emotional outbursts fall neatly into the category of strategies this chapter will discuss. Rather than making a direct effort to teach Jonas how to manage his emotions, they worked to structure all the external factors (the antecedents) to reduce the likelihood that he would become overloaded. Remember principle number 3 from Chapter 5? For Jonas's mom and dad, this turned out to be the "golden rule." They knew it was unrealistic at such a young age to expect Jonas to learn how to manage his emotions, so they structured his day so that his emotions were less likely to get out of control. They paid attention to all of the ways they could modify external factors (from principle number 4) but put a lot of emphasis on the social and physical environment.

The principle of starting with external modifications is so important—and so effective—because it removes the burden for decision making from the child. You don't ask your child to control her own behavior—nor are you teaching her to control her own behavior except, possibly, by way of example. You'll probably also find this approach easy to take because as parents you're already used to making environmental modifications as a way of managing a wide variety of immature behaviors. You erected physical barriers to keep the child who was just learning how to walk from falling downstairs, you placed fragile objects out of reach, and today you establish schedules to make sure your children get enough sleep, buy food that is healthy and restrict food intake to mealtimes or snack times, control the kind and amount of television your child can watch, and so forth. Now you're going to learn to address executive skill weaknesses in much the same way.

As we've explained, until your child's frontal lobes develop to the point where she can make good choices and good decisions, you as parents act as her frontal lobes, making those choices and decisions for the child. As your child matures—and the rate at which she will mature will not necessarily coincide with the rate at which other kids mature—you gradually transfer that decision-making process to the child. As you read in Chapter 5, your first efforts to respond to deficiencies in executive functioning are *external* to the child. You begin by altering the *environment* rather than altering the *child*. Over time, you'll transfer your efforts so that the child herself becomes a target for intervention. You do this by teaching your child skills, but even once you begin this teaching process, you're still moving in a progression from external to internal.

Back to Jonas: His parents addressed his weak emotional control with efforts that were completely external. Building in schedules and routines, modifying television viewing, reducing exposure to overstimulating events—none of these efforts were designed to teach Jonas to regulate his behavior or control his emotions. But they did make for a more smoothly functioning family because they reduced the likelihood that the events that triggered emotional upset in Jonas would occur. As Jonas gets older, his parents may begin to talk with him about what kinds of things upset him and what he can do to avoid them or cope with them when they occur. Increasing his understanding of his own behavior—when he is developmentally ready for it—will allow Jonas to begin adapting to his environment to meet his needs (for example, by voluntarily leaving a noisy family party and going off to his room to play alone for a while). It will also teach him how to cope with upsetting situations when they arise, such as by using self-soothing techniques or seeking an adult's help.

A wide variety of ways to modify or structure external factors to counteract the effect of weak or not-yet-developed executive skills are available to you, but they all fall into the three categories mentioned in principle number 4 in Chapter 5. You may find some of the following ideas familiar. Maybe you've used some of them without recognizing them as such. Or you've used them on and off but not religiously. If your child has ADHD, you may have already learned some behavior modification techniques. Please don't conclude there's nothing here for you if any of these are true for you. We're going to give you ways to use these strategies systematically, help you pick up the particular methods you may not have been using so far, and show you how you can zero in more specifically on the methods that will target your child's particular executive skill deficits instead of throwing the kitchen sink at random at them. For some kids, a more concerted effort to tweak the environment even in fairly basic ways is what's needed to give executive skill development a jumpstart. So please don't assume you've tried all this before and it hasn't been enough. You'll learn more about planning interventions for your child in Part III.

Change the Physical or Social Environment to Reduce Problems

These types of changes can take any number of forms depending on the executive skill weakness and the specific problem area. In terms of physical changes, children who have trouble with homework because of problems with task initiation, sustained attention, or time management often benefit from doing homework in the kitchen, where there are fewer distractions in the form of toys to play with and where parental supervision is more readily available. For a child with organizational problems that lead to messy bedrooms, limiting the number of toys she is allowed to keep in the bedroom or giving her bins or containers for each category of toy (with prominent labels) can facilitate bedroom cleaning. For children who are impulsive, parents should restrict access to settings, situations, or equipment that can lead to trouble. A child who may run out into the road to retrieve a ball is not allowed to play in the front yard. If a child throws things in anger, parents should keep expensive or breakable objects out of reach. For children who have difficulty waiting, parents can select restaurants where food is served fast, where the child is allowed to move around while waiting, or where activities to keep kids occupied are provided while they wait for their food.

Some children benefit from management of the social environment. For children with weak emotional control, this might include restricting the number of children coming over to play or the amount of time they will stay. For children who have difficulty with flexibility or impulse control, arranging for structured social activities such as playing organized games or going to the movies often works better than more open-ended play dates.

Here are a few of the ways that you can modify the physical or social environment:

• *Add physical barriers or make some locations off-limits.* Particularly for children with response inhibition problems, putting a fence around a yard or gates on stairs, placing breakable objects out of reach, locking rooms, such as Dad's tool shop, and taking away the controls to video games are all ways to control the physical environment. We know of parents with impulsive teenagers who hide car keys to ensure their children do not go for joy rides in the middle of the night, but that may be a more extreme example than most parents will need.

Also think about introducing barriers to technology as a way of managing executive skill problems. These include adding parental controls to cable television and video games (Xbox, for instance, offers parents the option of specifying the amount of time per day or per week children can play games; the game console shuts down when the limit is reached). Ways to control your child's use of the computer include the use of passwords to control access to the computer and/or to the Internet, as well as making use of filters to control what websites your children can visit. If you choose to let your kids go on social networking sites such as myspace or Facebook, make sure you know their passwords and check on their pages. Let your kids know you will be doing this—and do it regularly, including checking their history to see what websites they've been to.

• *Reduce distractions.* We've done workshops with middle school kids about homework where they've told us that one of the biggest obstacles to getting homework done is the noise that surrounds them at home. This may include a little brother watching cartoons in the late afternoon or an older brother blasting his stereo. Creating a "quiet time" for homework can increase your child's ability to focus on work and complete it efficiently. Other times when distractions need to be reduced may be at bedtime and during chores. Many young people use listening to music (for example, with iPods) as a way to screen out distractions; white noise generators (such as Bose headphones) are another way to block out distractions.

• *Provide organizational structures.* Remember that old expression *A place for everything and everything in its place*? It is certainly easier for children to develop organizational skills if organizational systems are in place. Providing cubbies and coat racks, storage bins for sports equipment and toys, and hampers in each bedroom for dirty clothes makes this a whole lot easier. And this is actually one example where, by prompting children to place belongings in their appropriate place, they will eventually (by the time they're 21 or 25!) internalize the concept of organization. You can also help shape organizational skills by letting kids know up front what level of organization is expected and how that expectation will be cued. For instance, take a photograph of what the final product should look like (as in a clean bedroom, playroom, etc.) so that you and your child together can compare her work to the photograph. Middle school students may benefit from using PDAs (personal digital assistants) to help them organize tasks or plan their time.

• *Reduce the social complexity of an activity or event.* Children who have problems with emotional control, flexibility, or response inhibition often struggle in complex social situations, such as when a lot of people are involved or the rules are loose.

Simplifying means keeping the number of people down or making the activity more structured. Keeping birthday parties small and ensuring there are carefully planned activities may make the difference between "a good time was had by all" and melt-downs. Open-ended social situations are particularly difficult for inflexible children to manage. In this case, the burden on the child can be reduced by having the activity dictate the social interaction (for example, watching a sporting event, movie or video, or visiting a museum or water park). Having clear rules for social situations and reminding children of the rules before the event begins can also help. Rules for play dates might include: *Play with one toy at a time, take turns,* and *no fighting.* By reminding your child and his friend what the rules are at the beginning of the play date, you're placing those rules in working memory so children are more likely to be able to retain and apply them.

• *Change the social mix.* While learning to live and work with all kinds of people is an important life lesson for children, there are times when it makes sense for parents to take charge and alter the social dynamics. There may be some children it's just not a good idea for your daughter to play with. Or maybe you've found that your son does great playing with more than one friend as long as one of those friends is not Joey (whom he does well with one-on-one). There's nothing wrong with structuring play dates or other social situations to avoid volatile combinations. Where it's not possible to do this (such as at family parties), anticipate having to provide more supervision than usual to avoid problems. We also recommend telling your child in advance what the default option is. For instance, you might say, "When I see you getting uncomfortable, this is what we're going to do." And be sure to provide a bail-out—a place the child or the parent can retreat to in the event of problems that's not embarrassing to either of them.

Change the Nature of the Tasks Your Child Is Expected to Perform

Many youngsters with executive skill problems do just fine as long as they're the ones deciding how to spend their time. They gravitate to tasks that are intrinsically appealing to them and stick with them as long as the tasks are fun. When they stop being fun, they shift to something else that *is* fun. This explains why summer vacation tends to be less stressful than the school year—because the ratio of fun to not-fun activities is stacked in favor of fun.

As parents, however, we all know that it's the rare individual indeed who gets to go through life doing only the fun stuff. To help prepare children for the adult world of work and family responsibilities, we expect them to tackle tasks that are not particularly appealing to them—whether it's doing chores or homework, going to boring family parties, or following schedules and routines. Many children can set aside their own preferences and do something they may not be particularly happy to do. Kids with executive skill weaknesses may not.

There are a wide variety of ways to ease the adjustment by modifying the tasks we are asking them to perform:

• *Make the task shorter.* For youngsters with problems with task initiation and sustained attention in particular, we generally say that when they begin the task *the end should be in sight.* For these youngsters in particular, it's better to ask them to do several brief tasks than to ask them to rake all the leaves in the backyard if your yard looks to them like Sherwood Forest.

• *If you do assign long tasks, build in frequent breaks.* If Sherwood Forest needs to be raked and there's no way around assigning your child to do it, break the task down. Have the child rake one section of lawn or rake for 15 minutes at a time rather than expecting him to do the whole lawn from start to finish.

• *Give the child something to look forward to when the task is done.* We'll talk about this in more detail in Chapter 8 when we talk about incentive systems, but one of the most powerful ways to alter how kids perceive the tasks we ask them to do is to hold out something fun for them to do when the dreaded task is finished.

• *Make the steps more explicit.* Rather than sending them to their bedroom with the assignment of "cleaning the whole room," break the task down into a series of subtasks. Very often, these subtasks can be turned into a checklist:

1. Put dirty clothes in laundry.
2. Place clean clothes in dresser drawers or on hangers in closet.
3. Put books on bookshelf.
4. Put toys in toy chest.

A similar approach can be used for things like morning or bedtime routines or any other chore that involves more than one step. We offer a whole chapter of daily routines broken down this way in Chapter 10.

• *Create a schedule for the child.* This is similar to making checklists, but it can be applied more broadly to help the day go more smoothly. Building in set times in the day when things such as mealtimes, bedtimes, chores, and homework occur not only lets children know what to expect, but also helps them internalize a sense of order and routine—prerequisite skills to help them develop more sophisticated planning, organization, and time management skills later on.

• *Build in choice or variety.* Rather than having children do the same chores day in and day out, creating a menu of chores and allowing them to choose which ones they want to do can make the tasks seem less aversive. You may also be able to let them choose when they want to do the chores, although this can get a little tricky— especially for children (or parents!) with weak working memory because they will likely require reminders for when they agreed to do the chores.

• *Make the task more appealing.* This might mean letting children complete the task with someone rather than alone or letting them listen to the radio or a favorite CD while they do the task. Some parents are very clever at turning chores into games. "See if you can finish your room before the timer goes off" can be a motivator, or "Let's place a bet—how many Lego pieces do you think are lying on your bedroom floor? I bet 100—what's your bet?" Other ways to turn chores into games include:

- Challenge your child to pick up 10 things in one minute.
- Schedule "fast clean" sessions. A teacher we know holds 15-minute "fast clean sessions" to get her students to help her tidy the classroom. This is followed by 15 minutes of free play.
- Turn picking up the playroom into a game like musical chairs. Start the music and have children wander around the playroom. When the music stops, children "freeze" and then pick up items within reaching distance of where they are standing.
- Write down chores to be done on pieces of paper, which are folded and put in a jar. Children select one piece of paper and perform the chore written on it.

Change the Way You (or Other Adults) Interact with the Child

The more you understand executive skills and the role they play in helping children become independent, the more you'll see how you can alter the way you interact with your child to promote executive skill development. Specifically, there are ways you can interact with your child *before*, *during*, and *after* situations that require executive functioning to increase the likelihood that the situation will go well either now or in the future.

What You Can Do before a Situation Comes Up

- *Rehearse with the child what will happen and how the child will handle it.*

Sara is going to her grandmother's for the afternoon. Sara's mom knows that her mother is a stickler for playing with toys one at a time and putting away the last toy before getting out the next one. So on the car ride over, she and Sara talk about how she will spend the afternoon and make an agreement that Sara will work on remembering to play with one toy at a time. Sara's mom tells Sara how pleased she will be if Sara is able to follow this rule because she knows it's important to Sara's grandmother.

Reviewing or rehearsing in advance can be used with any executive skill weakness, but it is particularly helpful with children who have problems with flexibility, emotional control, or response inhibition.

- *Use verbal prompts or reminders.* This is basically a shortened version of a rehearsal. "Remember what we talked about" will remind a child of a previous conversation in which rules were laid down or a situation previewed. Other examples might be: "What's the rule for playing in the front yard?" "What do you have to do before you get to call up Mike and invite him to come over?" "What do you have to do first as soon as you get home from school?" All of these examples, by the way, have one common characteristic: *they require the child to retrieve information*. You may ask, "What's the difference between telling my son he has to clean his room before he can call Mike and asking him what he has to do before calling Mike?" Here's the difference: by asking your son to retrieve the information himself, you're requiring him to begin to use his own executive skills, specifically *working memory*. This brings him just a little closer to independence. Of course, if he can't remember what he is supposed to do, you can help him out—but don't just say "Clean your room." Rather, give him the minimal amount of information necessary for him to answer the question. You might say, "Remember—we talked about it just before you went to bed last night." Or you might say, "Clean your . . . *what?*"

• *Arrange for other cues such as visual cues, written reminders, lists, audiotaped cues, alarms, or pager systems.* A sign on the kitchen table that says "Please walk the dog before you start playing video games" alerts the child with weak working memory what needs to be done when he gets home from school in the absence of his mother. Sometimes even more tangible reminders can be beneficial—having the child place his gym bag in front of the door so that he'll trip over it as he goes out to catch the bus is an example of this. Shopping lists, to-do lists, and vacation packing lists are all things adults use to remember large amounts of information. We have found that kids—especially those with executive skill problems—resist making lists or even referring to lists. To get your child accustomed to this, you can make the lists at first and prompt your child to "look at your list." Sooner or later, your child will realize how useful this strategy is and pick it up on her own. And thanks to modern technology, beepers and cell phones are readily available and relatively inexpensive. For youngsters with problems with working memory, task initiation, time management, and planning, you can use these remote signaling systems to prompt your child to do the tasks she needs to do—chores, homework, appointments, telephone calls she's promised to make, or whatever else goes into managing the complex details of growing up in 21st-century America. Over the years, parents and teachers we have worked with have recommended a number of these technological devises or services, such as Time Timers and WatchMinders (all have websites that are provided in the Resources section at the end of the book).

Ways You Can Interact with Your Child *during* an Activity or Problem Situation

• *Coach the child to elicit the rehearsed behavior.* A well-placed "Remember what we talked about" just before the problem is about to arise can make all the difference to a child with weak working memory or impulse control. You may even want to call a quick "Time out!" and remove the child from the situation briefly to go over that rehearsal again in a little more detail. We sometimes find it helpful to give kids "cue cards" that they can carry with them to remind them of the skill they're working on or how to carry out that skill. An example of a cue card for "Listening" is shown on page 90 (it also includes space to record when the child uses the skill).

- *Remind the child to check his list or schedule.* In the early phases of learning a routine or procedure, children forget not only that there is a procedure but also that it's been written down. A gentle reminder to them to check their list can get them back on track. And again, rather than telling them what step they're on and exactly what they have to do, prompting them to check the list aids the transfer of responsibility from parent to child.

- *Monitor the situation to better understand the triggers and other factors that affect your child's ability to use executive skills successfully.* Even when you can't intervene quickly enough or there's nothing you can do at the time to avert a problem, you can use your observational skills to identify the factors that contribute to problems. Being present during a problem situation may enable you to see how your older daughter cleverly "sets up" your younger daughter to lose her temper. Or you can see how the teasing your son got from older kids in the neighborhood led him to pick on his little sister when he came in for supper. Of course, you can't always be there to see what causes problems to arise, but when you do happen to be present, if you can step back and think about it objectively, you may learn a lot about how to handle the same situation differently in the future.

What You Can Do Afterward to Improve Your Child's Use of Executive Skills the Next Time Around

- *Praise your child for using good skills.* "I like the way you started your homework with only one reminder from me," "Thank you for showing self-control when your brother teased you," and "I was impressed with the way you were able to set aside your video games without complaining when it was time for you to start your chores" are all examples of ways you can reinforce effective use of executive skills. This will be discussed in more detail in Chapter 8.

- *Debrief.* This means reviewing the situation to see if lessons can be learned. Talk with your child about what happened, what worked or didn't work, and what might be done differently the next time. This tactic needs to be used judiciously. Debriefing should be done at some distance from the incident to avoid arousing all over again the bad feelings associated with the problem event. It should also be used sparingly. We've known parents concerned about their children's difficulty making friends who felt they needed to debrief after every social encounter. This had the effect of heightening their child's anxiety around social contacts rather than helping her learn better ways of connecting with other kids. When it *is* used judiciously, however, debriefing can be "the teachable moment."

- *Consult with others involved in the situation.* This might mean asking for feedback from a spouse who observed the event and might be able to offer useful insight

CUE CARD FOR LISTENING

Week of:	Monday		Tuesday		Wednesday		Thursday		Friday	
Who? When?										
Face speaker										
Pay attention and show interest										
Keep body still										
Do not interrupt										
Overall rating of entire skill performance										

+ = independent/successful; h = with help; − = did not use skill or did incorrectly.

into what happened. Or it might mean making a suggestion to a babysitter about how to handle the situation differently next time. In other words, consulting with others can give you the opportunity to change your own behavior or make suggestions to others for changing what they do to make things go more smoothly the next time.

As we said at the outset, modifying the environment does not require the child to change. However, many of the strategies we've described will, over time, help children internalize procedures that will facilitate the development of their own executive skills. In some cases, time and patience may be what's needed. The question is how long you can afford to wait. If your child is falling behind in school or suffering in other ways from lack of executive skills, you may want to combine environmental modifications with direct instruction, as described in the next chapter. You can modify external factors, put interventions in place to address particularly problematic tasks, tackle a whole executive skill (or two or three) in all of the domains in which the child interacts, use scaffolding and games to give your child a more organic type of boost, provide incentives (or, less preferably, penalties) for using executive skills, or choose any combination of these interventions. It all depends on the severity of the child's problems and how much time you can invest. You'll read about all these options starting in the next chapter and then through Part III.

7

....

Teaching Executive Skills Directly
B Is for *Behavior*

Noriko, age 8, had a horrible time getting ready for school in the morning. It took her forever to get dressed, she dawdled over breakfast, and she became absorbed with the television when she should have been brushing her teeth and combing her hair. Her mother felt like a broken record getting her through the morning routine: "Noriko, find your shoes, Noriko, wash your face, Noriko, get your backpack so I can put your lunch in it." As she listened to her own voice, Noriko's mother hated the way she sounded, but she knew without constant prompts and reminders Noriko would miss the bus. Finally she decided something had to change. She and Noriko sat down one night after dinner and made a list of the things she had to do to get ready for school in the morning. Noriko was a talented artist, so her mother had her draw a small picture for each step in the morning routine. Her mother took the pictures to the school she worked at and used the laminating machine to cover each picture in plastic. She bought Velcro and she and Noriko worked together to attach a small strip to the back of each picture and to a poster board cut to fit all the pictures. She divided the poster board into two columns labeled TO DO and DONE! She explained to Noriko that from now on she was not going to tell her what to do in the morning, but she was going to remind her to check her picture schedule. Each time she finished a task, she got to move the laminated card from the TO DO column to the DONE! column. If Noriko was able to finish the list with more than 15 minutes left before the bus came, she would be allowed to turn on the television and watch cartoons until it was time to go to the bus stop. After several weeks of reminders to Noriko to check her list, Noriko began to complete her morning routine by herself. Her mom marveled at how much more smoothly everything went—she even had time to enjoy a cup of coffee while Noriko watched television.

The previous chapter focused on ways to modify the environment (the antecedents) to reduce the impact of weak executive skills. That's often the easiest way to tackle the problems associated with weak executive skills, and it's particularly appropriate for the youngest kids—which is why Chapter 6 opened with an example involving a 4-year-old. The trouble is, environmental interventions are not portable. If this is all you've got in your parental repertoire, you're going to have to ensure that modifications are instituted in every environment the child is in. That's hard enough when you're with the child, but expecting to be able to prevail on the adults in charge at school, church, Scouts, the athletic field, or a friend's house to take this trouble is unrealistic.

The alternative is to work with children to help them develop better-functioning executive skills. We do this in one of two ways: Either by teaching the skills we want them to have or by motivating them to practice using the skills they have but don't use much. We generally encourage parents to use both, so you might want to read this chapter along with Chapter 8 before deciding what approaches to take with your child. Noriko's mother used instruction and motivation to help her daughter get through a difficult time of day—she taught her a set of steps to follow, and she arranged for a reward (television) if Noriko was able to get through her morning routine in an efficient manner. The next chapter will talk about strategies that can be used to motivate children to use or practice executive skills. For now, let's focus on how we teach these skills.

There are two different ways to teach your child executive skills:

1. You can do so naturally and informally by how you respond to your child's behavior and how you talk to your child throughout life beginning in toddlerhood and also by using games that encourage the development of various executive skills.
2. You can take a more targeted approach and teach your child how to manage certain problematic tasks involving executive skills that you know your child lacks to some degree.

We'll explain how to do both in this chapter. Many parents do, in fact, choose to do both. Scaffolding and games are a great way to "sneak in" valuable instruction kind of in the same way you might sneak all kinds of healthy nutrients into a child's diet by making "milk shakes" full of fruit and yogurt. The child receives valuable lessons in developing and using executive skills outside of the conflict-ridden domain of chores and other undesirable activities. Meanwhile, you can target one or two routine tasks that are really causing trouble for everyone and design a specific intervention for teaching your child to do that job and acquire the necessary executive skills. (Or you can use the interventions we've already designed for a long list of the typically troublesome routines in a family's life; see Chapter 10.)

Teaching Executive Skills Informally

Research shows that children whose mothers employ "verbal scaffolding" with them at age 3 tend to have better problem-solving skills and goal-directed behavior (that is, executive skills) at age 6 than children whose mothers don't use this technique. What do we mean by *scaffolding*? Providing explanations and guidance and asking questions at an appropriate developmental level for the child. It's actually another way of saying *provide just enough support necessary for the child to be successful*, with an emphasis on helping children understand relationships, make connections between concepts, or connect new learning to prior knowledge. The more skillfully children can do all these things—see patterns, make connections, and draw on past knowledge—the easier it is for them to create plans or organizational schemes. Even more directly, these skills form the underpinning of *metacognition*, that more complex executive skill that involves using thought in the service of problem solving. The more extensive the background knowledge children have and the more practice they've had building up that knowledge and connecting new information to known information, the easier it will be for them to access that information and use it for different purposes, including making plans, organizing material, and solving problems.

Verbal Scaffolding

Verbal scaffolding is a deceptively powerful strategy that parents often apply instinctively with the youngest children, perhaps because the rewards are so immediately evident. Seeing the pride on the face of a 2-year-old as she points to pictures of animals you name while you look at a book together or holds up the correct number of fingers when asked how old she is just naturally makes us want to keep up this type of scaffolding. Turning meal preparation and other chores and errands into a game for a young child can make the time pass enjoyably for parent and child. Unfortunately, many parents today find themselves talking less to their children and relying on TV and other devices to keep kids occupied while Mom and Dad try to get more and more done in less and less time. If you find yourself in that bind, keep in mind that verbal scaffolding can be used in a variety of contexts over the course of the day—when getting dressed in the morning, at the dinner table, remarking on things you see on the drive to school or daycare, when watching television programs, and in the context of the kinds of play activities your child enjoys. (See the examples of verbal scaffolding appropriate when talking with preschoolers in the table on p. 95.) You'll probably be pleased to see how much you're already building your child's

Using Scaffolding with Preschoolers

Scaffolding category	Example
Questions/statements that associate objects with location	"Which piece goes here?" (pointing to a place on a puzzle). "Where is the shirt that goes with those shorts?"
Relating current activity, object, or topic of conversation to a previous experience	"That's a giraffe. You saw one at the zoo." "It's like making cookies" (e.g., when playing with Play-Doh).
Using words to describe experiences, especially focusing on sensory descriptions	"It tastes spicy." "That whistle sounds like a blue jay."
Describing characteristics for an object that identifies its uniqueness or use, function, or specific features that can be used for problem solving	"It's not the same color" (for an activity where color matching is required). "Hit the nail. It's the one that's round on top."
Specifying the function or activity that could be done with the object	"Check the baby's temperature" (handing the child a thermometer). "That's what you use to blow your nose" (child holding a tissue).
Verbalizing while physically demonstrating how to do something	"This is how you roll the car." "This is how you open the jar."
Associating feelings or emotions with a reason for the emotions	"Your brother is crying because he wants the ball." "She will get angry if you take that away from her."
Teaching cause and effect or what you need to do to make something work	"You need to wear shoes if you're going outside because it's too cold to go barefoot." "If you bear down too hard, you'll break the pencil lead."
Linking specific objects with general categories	"Look at all the animals—a dog, a cat, a bear." "There is furniture in your doll house. Here's a chair and a table."
Helping the child understand activities by linking two aspects of the activity	"We need a cake if we are going to have a birthday party." "Let's play ring around the rosie. Give me your hand."

Adapted from Landry, S. H., Miller-Loncar, C. L., Smith, K. E., & Swank, P. R. (2002). The role of early parenting in children's development of execute processes. *Developmental Psychology, 21,* 15–41. Copyright by Taylor & Francis Group. Adapted with permission.

executive skills with this type of scaffolding—and possibly feel motivated to do even more.

The more you can help children think about what they do and why—or think about the dangers associated with some actions and behaviors—the more they will be able to use that thinking in any problem-solving situation. Children who understand how certain events trigger certain feelings are more likely to gain control over their emotions or curtail their impulses. The more they understand a cause-and-effect sequence, the better they'll be able to plan a course of action. And when you explain why something is important, your children are more likely to remember that critical information when they need it. Of course, explanations alone are generally insufficient to help children acquire better-functioning executive skills—but instruction that lacks explanation is unlikely to be very effective.

Some other verbal-scaffolding ways to infuse executive skill instruction into activities of daily living are:

• *Ask, don't tell.* Examples: "Why do I ask you to wash your hands before dinner? What would happen if I let you stay up as long as you wanted at night? How do you think you could remember to give your teacher the permission slip?"

• *Explain rather than dictate.* Sometimes we parents rely on direct commands and explicit instructions that emphasize the power differential between ourselves and our children: "Just do what I say!" or "Because I said so!" This is understandable. We get tired. Our minds are occupied with other things, and we feel we don't have the time or energy to stop and think about how to phrase an explanation appropriate for our child's age and abilities. Or, sometimes accurately, we suspect asking for a reason is a stall tactic on the part of the child. But even if it is, dictating is less likely to foster the development of executive skills than an approach that emphasizes the reason for something. Remember, first and foremost, executive skills are the skills we use to execute tasks. The more we understand about a given situation—cause and effect, why something is important, why something has to be done in a certain way, and so forth—the more we can use that information either to design our own task execution process or motivate ourselves to use the process laid out for us by someone else. "If you don't take your medicine, your strep throat will come back" or "If you leave your bicycle outdoors, it will get rusty when it rains tonight" are examples of this approach. Explanations largely build the skill of metacognition, but they enhance working memory too. We remember things better when we have a reason for remembering. If someone says to you, "Don't forget to take your passport with you to the airport, or they won't let you on the plane to Jamaica and you'll miss out on your vacation," aren't you more likely to remember your passport than if someone says, "Don't forget to take your passport to the airport"? The same goes for your child. This approach, of course, should be used judiciously. Some children do attempt to avoid tasks by asking for endless explanations for why they need to do something. Answer the question the first time they ask and then don't engage them further.

- *Let your child know you understand how she's feeling and why.* "You're disappointed because you were really counting on going over to Jane's house and now it can't happen today." "You're worried that you're going to make a mistake on your speech and everyone will laugh at you."

- *Encourage self-appraisal.* When you give solutions, pass judgment, or tell your child what to do differently the next time, you're depriving him of being able to do this thinking for himself. "What can you do to get out of this jam?" "How do you think you did on your Scout project?" "What do you think you might do differently the next time so your friend doesn't ask to go home early?"

Using Games to Help Your Child Develop Executive Skills

Games are another natural, informal way to help children develop executive skills. Even classic games like checkers, Chinese checkers, and chess require planning, sustained attention, response inhibition, working memory, and metacognition among others. The simplest of board games like Candyland require attention, response inhibition, and goal-directed persistence for young children, while games like Monopoly and Clue additionally involve planning and working memory. Battleship requires attention, planning and organization, inhibition, and metacognition. Holding family game nights and encouraging your child to play such games with siblings and friends is always a good idea.

For the many kids who find video games more appealing than the board games more familiar to parents and grandparents, we can mention a few representative examples that help build executive skills. Most of these fall into some type of strategy/problem-solving category. For younger children, Webkinz involves care of a "pet." Across a wider age range, the Legend of Zelda, Simcity and its variations, and Command and Conquer all require sustained attention, response inhibition, planning, organization, metacognition, and goal-directed persistence. Naturally, the content varies in age appropriateness, but you'll probably know what games your child's peers are playing. Video game demos and previews can be seen at Game Revolution, GameSpot, or GameSpy on the Internet. Video game ratings are available at the Electronic Software Ratings Board, Common Sense Media, and Family Media Guide. The PTA has a PTA/ESRB Brochure on Video Game Safety that provides tips for parents about games and monitoring.

In a category of its own, managing fantasy sports teams has become popular and for children interested, this "game" involves most of the above-noted executive skills along with task initiation and time management.

You can even build executive skills with time-honored games like tic tac toe, hangman, and twenty questions when you're waiting in the doctor's office, taking a car trip, or waiting for your order at a restaurant.

We should note that while all of these activities can enhance executive skills, there is little research on how well skills learned in these activities transfer to real-world situations. At this point, it is an open question. Transfer is more likely if you can help your child see how a skill learned in one situation can be used in another (for example, parent to child: "Brad, before we think about a pet, let's figure out what we would need to have").

Teaching Executive Skills in the Course of Family Activities

Another way to build executive skills that's fun and motivating is to teach them in the context of real-world family activities like meal planning, cooking, grocery shopping, clothes shopping, vacation planning, and banking. Here we're not talking about assigning chores but enlisting children as participants in activities that are important to the family. These activities can be ideal teaching tools because they have built-in incentives (you get to buy or eat what you chose, put money in the bank, or do something fun on vacation). Beyond that, they offer a range of options for participation (from adding an ingredient to preparing a meal) and for degree of independence. While they can be done at any age, starting young is recommended because children are more likely to be excited about the choices and less likely to see the activity as a chore.

There are a few important considerations to keep in mind if these activities are to be effective in promoting executive skills:

- *You have to be an active and available participant in order to model the skills, ask key questions, and encourage the child.* In other words, you need to be a good frontal lobe. You can't just invite your child to join in the planning and then leave her to her own devices.
- *The child must have some legitimate choices and decision-making power in the activity.* If the family doesn't end up preparing the meal that the child participated in planning, if you don't buy the items on the grocery list compiled, or if you say you're allowing the child to choose vacation activities but then reject all of his ideas, the child will lose interest. That means that before you enlist your child's help you have to decide what choices you can live with. If "junk food" is not an option on the grocery list or for cooking, make sure the child knows that ahead of time. Work up a list of exclusions before the brainstorming begins. Or make it clear that your child can't pick the vacation location but can help plan an activity.
- Be prepared to accurately gauge your child's interest, attention span, and endurance and provide enough support so that the child is successful in and appreciated for whatever job she does. To help with attention and interest, let your child know, a little in advance if possible, you would appreciate her help in deciding some details about the meal, shopping list, vacation, etc. ("Ashley, after you're finished playing, could you help me with . . . ?"). Pick a time when she is not already engaged in some other activity of interest and ask if it's a good time. For younger children especially, keep the activity short, the choices concrete, and at the first sign of fading attention or lack of interest, thank the child and end it. Later, when the choice has been acted on, acknowledge it to family, friends, or whoever else is around ("Ashley helped/decided the menu tonight"). Older children may be willing to offer

more time or may seek more involvement (like finding recipes, managing the meal, searching for vacation options). As long as the available options are clear, encourage them to be as involved in the process as they want.

Direct Interventions for Teaching Executive Skills

All of the informal approaches discussed so far can be very helpful to your child, but chances are, if you've picked up this book and read this far, you have a child with a specific skill deficit that requires a more direct intervention. What follows is an instructional sequence that can be used for teaching all kinds of behaviors (not just the ones we're focusing on in this book). It forms the framework for the interventions we've designed for specific routine tasks in Chapter 10 and for designing your own aimed at particular executive skills in Chapters 11–21.

Step 1: Identify the Problem Behavior You Want to Work On

This may sound easier than it is. The more frustrated you are with your child, the more likely you are to refer to problem behaviors in global terms that do not describe specific actions. When we say a child is *lazy, irresponsible, a slob,* or *just doesn't care,* the words do communicate something about the child in question, but they really don't give us a starting point for teaching executive skills. Helpful descriptions are those that depict behaviors that can be seen or heard. They also identify when or under what circumstances the problems occur. Here are some examples:

- Whines and complains when it's time to do homework.
- Doesn't complete chores unless someone's there to remind him.
- Leaves personal belongings all over the house.
- Rushes through homework, resulting in messy work and careless mistakes.

Why is it important to define the problem behavior? Because it helps you clarify what it is, exactly, you're going to teach. Teaching someone not to be a slob sounds like a thankless, if not impossible, task. Teaching a child to keep his personal belongings off the living room floor is a more achievable goal. Which brings us to the next step in the instructional sequence.

Step 2: Set a Goal

The goal, very often, is a positive restatement of the problem behavior. A goal says what the child is expected to do using terms that describe behaviors that can be seen or heard. Using the problem behaviors described above, the goals might be:

- Starts homework without complaining.
- Completes chores on time without reminders.

- Takes personal belongings out of living room before going to bed.
- Completes homework neatly with a minimum of mistakes.

Sometimes it may be sufficient for you to set a goal in a rather informal way and just tuck it into the back of your mind. *By the time my son graduates from high school I sure hope he'll be able to pick up his bedroom by himself might fall into that category.* For intractable—and important—executive skill deficits, however, it can be helpful to be more overt and explicit. Remembering to bring home sports equipment and to take homework to school are examples of goals we want to work on with our children very directly.

Involve Your Child in Goal Setting

When goals fall into this category, we find it helpful to involve children in the goal-setting process rather than dictating to them what we expect them to do. You've probably noticed that this idea falls right in line with the ideas we offered in the scaffolding discussion earlier in this chapter: anything that encourages participation and independent, critical thinking fosters executive skills. In the scenario that began this chapter, Noriko's mother sat down with her and discussed the problem. She enlisted her help in recognizing that the problem was real and keeping both of them from having a smooth start to the day. She may have said something like "Noriko, how does it make you feel when I'm always bugging you to do things in the morning?" And maybe Noriko said, "It puts me in a bad mood." At that point, her mother would have been able to say, "What do you say we try to come up with a plan to make the morning go more smoothly?"

Set Interim Goals

Determining the final outcome is important to the skill-teaching process, but you won't get there right away. So you'll have to set and accept interim goals along the way. Starting homework without reminders may be the final goal, but in the early stages you may need to live with a goal of starting homework with no more than three reminders.

How do you know what a reasonable interim goal is? Ideally, you take a baseline—you measure the current behavior and set as a first interim goal something that's a slight improvement on the current behavior. So if you find that it generally takes five or six reminders for your daughter to get started on her homework, maybe getting started with no more than three or four reminders is a reasonable first step.

When we say "measure the current behavior," we really do mean *measure*. In the example above, we mean *count* the number of times the behavior occurs. Examples of ways to measure are:

- *Time how long it takes between the time a child says she will start something and the time she actually starts* (as in, "Sarah has agreed to start her homework every night at

7 o'clock. Before putting in place an intervention, her mother times her for a week to see how much later than 7 o'clock she actually begins").

● *Time how long something lasts* (as in, "Joey says he will spend 30 minutes every day practicing his trumpet. His mother doesn't think he lasts that long, so she measures how long he actually practices so she has some data to point to when she talks with him about the problem").

● *Count the number of times the behavior occurs.* This could either be positive behaviors (as in the number of days your child remembered to hand in all her homework) or problem behaviors (as in the number of meltdowns your 4-year-old has in the course of a day). If the number of behaviors is relatively small, you can count them all day long. If the behavior occurs frequently, then choose a part of the day to focus on (as in the number of complaints your child utters in the hour before dinner).

● *Count the number of reminders you need to give your child before she does what you've asked her to do.*

● *Create a 5-point scale and rate the severity of the problem behavior.* If your son has a problem managing stress or anxiety, a 5-point scale to measure his anxiety level that you and he could use to measure this might look like:

1—I'm doing fine.
2—I'm getting a little worried.
3—Now I'm nervous.
4—I'm feeling really upset.
5—I might lose control!

For further suggestions for how to use a 5-point scale, we recommend the book *The Incredible 5-Point Scale* by Kari Dunn Buron and Mitzi Curtis.

These kinds of baseline data are often most useful when you can display the results visually. An example of this can be seen in the graph on page 102.

If taking a baseline and setting precise goals are more than you want to attempt, though, you should shoot for "some improvement" as an interim goal. As time goes on, if you think you're not getting that improvement, you may want to back up and consider taking some more precise measures so you know for sure whether that's the case.

Step 3: Outline the Steps the Child Needs to Follow to Reach the Goal

In Part III we will provide lots of examples of this, using the kinds of problem situations that parents report to us are the most frustrating. But returning to Noriko, she and her mother made a list of the different tasks she had to do before leaving the house to catch the school bus in the morning. Other skills, like learning to manage emotions, control impulses, or handle frustration, may be a little more challenging

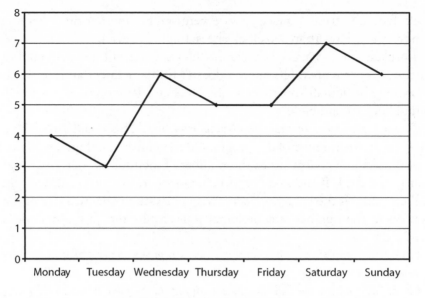

Reminders to do chores.

to think about using this procedure, but, again, we'll give you examples of how this might work in Part III.

Step 4: Turn the Steps into a List, a Checklist, or a Short Set of Rules to Be Followed

This accomplishes several things. First of all, it forces you to think clearly, logically, and succinctly about the skill you're trying to teach. Second, it creates a permanent record of the instructional sequence that you and your child can refer to so you can remember the process. Third, by checking off each item in the list, your child has the satisfaction of recording his progress toward a goal. The act of checking off items as they are completed serves as intermediate reinforcers on the road to the larger goal (task completion or a reward that may come with task completion). Finally, it builds in accountability—it's a way of documenting that the child is actually doing what he agreed to do.

Noriko and her mother made a picture schedule for Noriko to follow, but another way to deal with helping children follow morning routines might be to create a checklist such as the one shown on page 103. This checklist includes a column where you can check off how many reminders each step in the sequence required. This would be useful in situations where the biggest source of frustration to you is the number of reminders your child requires to get through her morning routine. After a week of using a checklist like this, progress will be readily apparent—as will the trouble spots (that is, which steps in the sequence require the greatest number of reminders). A copy of this checklist is included in Chapter 10 (pp. 132–135). A blank general-purpose checklist is also included at the end of this chapter for those of you who want to create your own checklist to cover the particular skill sequence you want to teach.

Task	Number of reminders Tally marks (/ / / /)	Done (✓)
MORNING ROUTINE CHECKLIST		
Get up		
Get dressed		
Eat breakfast		
Brush teeth		
Brush hair		
Get backpack ready for school		

From *Smart but Scattered* by Peg Dawson and Richard Guare. Copyright 2009 by The Guilford Press.

Before we leave this step, let's talk about a different kind of skill we want to teach children. Let's say 12-year-old Todd has a problem with emotional control. It shows up in lots of different situations, but what drives his dad crazy is how quickly he melts down when he encounters an obstacle during homework. It can happen for almost any kind of homework, but his dad has noticed that math seems to be the worst. He decides to talk to Todd about better ways of managing his frustration around math. Todd's father is smart enough to know that having this conversation in the middle of a meltdown is not likely to go well, so he waits until the end of a homework session that went smoothly for Todd. He starts the conversation with his son by remarking on how well this session went compared to some others and asks Todd why this might be. Todd says, "Yeah, I knew exactly what to do. I remembered the way Mr. Frank told us how to do the homework. I get mad when I can't remember—or when I think I remember but it doesn't work out right."

Todd's dad asks him if he knows before he even starts that the homework's going to be a problem, or if it's only once he's started working. Todd says, "Both—but what really makes me mad is when I thought I could do it but then I couldn't."

With a lot of sympathy and what psychologists call "reflective listening" (mirroring back the child's feelings, as in "That makes you so mad you want to throw your math book against the wall, huh?"), Todd's father was able to get Todd to consider whether there were things he could do to help him manage the frustration more successfully. Todd finally agreed that when he felt himself getting mad during math homework he would do two things. The first thing he would do would be to walk away from the problem for a few minutes. Quite literally—he agreed to get up from the desk in his bedroom and walk downstairs to the family room where he was likely to find his dad reading the newspaper. If clearing his head didn't resolve the problem for him (and Todd admitted that doing that sometimes helped him remember how to do the work), then Todd agreed to ask his dad for help. The rules for managing math could be boiled down to two words: *walk* and *talk*. His dad took an index card and wrote on it:

Math Lifeline

1. Walk
2. Talk

He taped the index card to Todd's desk as a reminder.

Step 5: Supervise the Child Following the Procedure

Here what's critical is understanding that children cannot be expected to learn a new skill after a single exposure to the steps involved. That would be like assuming that a child can follow all the rules of baseball after the first T-ball practice. Children require ongoing support and supervision as they perform the new skill, and this support needs to be provided as a matter of course and without resentment on the part of the parent.

We recommend beginning this step by holding a practice session or two—what might be called a "dry run." Once Noriko and her mom finished making the picture schedule, her mom said, "Let's try it out." She and Noriko walked through the steps, beginning with Noriko lying on her bed and pretending to sleep and her mother coming in and saying (as only mothers can), "Rise and shine, Noriko." Noriko then jumped out of bed, went to where her schedule sat on the bureau in her bedroom, and moved the "wake-up" picture from the TO DO to the DONE! column. She then pretended to get dressed and moved the second picture on the schedule, and then pretended her way through to the end of the list.

Noriko and her mom were now ready for the first real-life test of the process. For the first week or so, her mom had to remind her about using the schedule. Her mom found, happily, that as she moved each picture to the DONE! column, that step prompted Noriko to look at the next picture on the list, so that the reward (moving the picture) naturally led to the next step in the sequence, and before long her mom no longer needed to prompt Noriko at all.

It was a little harder for Todd's father to persuade Todd to go through a practice session to rehearse the frustration management procedure. Todd, after all, was on the edge of adolescence and thought that kind of role-play was "silly." So his dad decided the way to start was to model the procedure himself as if he were Todd. And he deliberately injected some humor into the process to pull Todd in. He muttered a few made-up curse words at the math book, picked it up as if to heave it at the wall, and then stopped himself in midthrow. "Oh, wait!" he said, and now his voice became sarcastic. "Dad wants me to walk downstairs. Okay, I'll do it, but I won't like it." He was successful enough in his role-play that Todd was willing to create his own humorous version of the skit. They played it two different ways—once where the walk downstairs was enough to get Todd back on track and once where he had to ask his dad for help. With these rehearsals under his belt, the first time he really had to use the process didn't feel as strange to Todd as his father feared it would. Before beginning math homework each night, though, for the first couple of weeks his dad said to him, "Okay, Todd, what's the plan when you find yourself getting mad?" After a while, Todd's father noticed that he was using the same process on other frustrating homework.

Step 6: Fade the Supervision

This is basically a reiteration of the last two principles described in Chapter 5. Mistakes are often made in failing to provide adequate support long enough for the child to acquire the skill and in failing to reduce the supports gradually.

Here's an example of how fading works. Thirteen-year-old Molly is now in seventh grade. She's in a new school where the homework load is considerably greater than it was in sixth grade, in part because she is changing classes for the first time and teachers don't seem to coordinate the homework they assign. When the first marking period progress report came out, Molly's parents learned that she was missing a number of homework assignments and was in danger of failing a couple of classes as a result. When they talked with Molly about this, she said, "I can't keep track of everything I have to do. I keep forgetting stuff!" After talking with her homeroom teacher, her parents found that classroom teachers were required to post all homework assignments on the school website. They made a deal with Molly that her daily homework session would begin with her checking the website and making a plan. Together they developed a form she would complete in which she listed each subject she had homework in and when she planned to start the assignment (a homework Daily Planner form is included in Chapter 10, p. 152, and also at the end of this chapter). They also put in a column for her to check off when she finished the assignment.

In the beginning, Molly and her mom filled out the form together in the late afternoon as soon as her mom got home from work. She needed reminders to start her homework at the agreed-upon time and to use the form to check off each assignment as she finished it. Gradually, her mother found she could back off on the amount of prompting and supervision required. The box below lists the steps she followed in fading the supervision. By the end of seventh grade, Molly continued to check the website each day to make sure she hadn't forgotten anything, but homework completion had become enough of a routine that apart from making a brief list of the tasks she had to do, she no longer needed to keep a more detailed planner.

Steps for Fading Supervision

Level of Independence in Planning Homework

- Filled in form with assistance; needed prompts to use form while completing homework.
- Needed prompt to use form and monitoring throughout process.
- Needed prompt to use form and check-in when done.
- Needed prompt to use form; no check-in required at end.
- Used form independently without prompt.

So What Does the Teaching Process Look Like?

Let's put the whole process together using as an example another very common childhood responsibility: room cleaning. Much as it takes time for language to develop in children, it also takes time for them to learn how to clean their rooms independently. In the beginning, parents who decide to teach their children how to clean their rooms act as their children's frontal lobes. And what do frontal lobes do?

- They provide a plan, an organizational scheme, and a specific set of directions.
- They monitor performance.
- They provide encouragement/motivation and feedback about the success of the approach.
- They problem solve when something doesn't work.
- They determine when the task is completed.

Thus, *Stage 1* in teaching room cleaning is very parent directed. Here are things parents might say to children as they supervise the process:

- "Let's start now."
- "Put your trucks in this box."
- "Put your dirty clothes in the laundry."
- "Put your books on the bookshelf."
- "There are two toys under the bed."
- "It doesn't look like all those toys will fit in that one box; we'll need to get another one."
- "When you finish, you can play with your friends."
- "I know you hate doing this, but you're almost done, and then you'll feel great!"
- "Isn't it nice to have all your work for the day done?"

Steps for Designing a Direct Intervention to Teach Executive Skills

1. Identify the problem behavior you want to work on.
2. Set a goal.
   - Involve the child in goal setting.
   - Set interim goals.
3. Outline the steps the child needs to follow to reach the goal.
4. Turn the steps into a list, a checklist, or a short list of rules to be followed.
5. Supervise the child following the procedure.
6. Fade the supervision.

At *Stage 2*, parents provide the same information without being the direct agent. They create a list, a picture schedule, or an audiotape to cue the child. At this stage, rather than tell the child what to do, parents say *Look at your list.*

At *Stage 3*, parents step back a little more. Rather than tell the child to look at the list, they may say, "What do you need to do?" By asking rather than telling, and making the questions somewhat vague, they force the child to do some problem solving on his own (or at least retrieve from his own working memory what needs to happen next).

At *Stage 4*, the transfer is now complete. The child may wake up on Saturday morning, look around his messy room, and say to himself, "What do I need to do?" Of course, by now the child may actually be a teenager or a young adult! Sometimes it takes a long time for children to internalize this kind of process.

Don't despair. Kids do learn—and the process may speed up (or at least stay on track) if you make sure they're motivated. That's the subject of the next chapter.

CHECKLIST

Task	Number of reminders Tally marks (/ / / /)	Done (✓)

From *Smart but Scattered* by Peg Dawson and Richard Guare. Copyright 2009 by The Guilford Press.

DAILY HOMEWORK PLANNER

Date: _____

Subject/assignment	Do I have all the materials?	Do I need help?	Who will help me?	How long will it take?	When will I start?	Done (✓)
	Yes ☐ No ☐	Yes ☐ No ☐				
	Yes ☐ No ☐	Yes ☐ No ☐				
	Yes ☐ No ☐	Yes ☐ No ☐				
	Yes ☐ No ☐	Yes ☐ No ☐				
	Yes ☐ No ☐	Yes ☐ No ☐				
	Yes ☐ No ☐	Yes ☐ No ☐				

8

··

Motivating Your Child to Learn and Use Executive Skills

C Is for Consequence

The parents of 3-year-old Melissa are just beginning to get her to think about picking up after herself. As part of her bedtime ritual, she and her mom or dad work together to pick up her playroom. As they work, her parents use words of encouragement to keep her going ("We've put the puzzles away; now we just have to pick up your dolls"), and when they're done, they praise her for helping. They realize how well this works when Melissa begins to praise herself. "I'm a hard worker, aren't I, Daddy?" Melissa says one night before her father has a chance to tell her the same thing.

Raj, age 9, loves video games. He could spend hours playing them, and his parents have found they have to limit the amount of time he plays to ensure he gets exercise and fresh air. When he goes back to school in the fall, his parents tell Raj they're concerned about how much time he spends on video games and how much less exercise he gets. They ask him what might be done about this. Together, they agree on a new rule: no more than 1 hour per night of video games, and he can't play unless he's had some active outdoor time. Later, when Raj finds there's a video game that builds in exercise, they amend the rule to allow him every other day to count the exercise video game as his hour of exercise.

Logan is 13 and has always been an avid skier. Recently, however, he's seen all his friends take up snowboarding, and he thinks he'd really like to get into that, too. All last winter he hassled his parents about buying him not just any snowboard but a top-of-the-line board so he could start snowboarding competitively.

Since the beginning of middle school, Logan's parents have been worried about his attitude toward school. They're afraid he's becoming an indifferent student despite being bright and wanting to attend college, so his parents decide they have to do something to encourage him to work harder at his studies. At the beginning of eighth grade, they talk with Logan about their concerns. They tell him they know that because he's an active kid who hates to sit down and study, they're willing to make a deal with him if he can think of something he might be willing to work for. Logan reminds them of the snowboard he really wants to get before winter. Together they hammer out an agreement that Logan will shoot for grades of B– or better on tests and quizzes. If in any given week he gets no more than one C on a test or quiz, he will earn 20 points. For every grade of B+ or better, he gets 5 more points. If he has 300 points by Christmas, his parents agree to buy him the snowboard he wants as a Christmas present. It took a little effort to get his teachers to agree to communicate with them regularly about Logan's test grades, but they simplified it by having teachers email them only if Logan earned grades of C or worse. To earn the extra points, Logan had to produce the test or quiz as proof of the grade. Because Logan's grades improved quickly, this placed little burden on his teachers.

These three scenarios depict different ways you can use motivational strategies to help your child develop executive skills. Sometimes, as in the case of Melissa, it can be as simple as remembering to say something positive about the child's behavior. Or, as in the case of Raj, it can mean just ensuring that the child does the have-to before getting to the want-to. Sometimes, we admit, motivational strategies have to be a little more elaborate, as in the case of Logan, where a careful plan and monitoring were required.

Motivation is important whether you're trying to get your child to stick to the sequence of rules or steps in an intervention you've designed or just trying to encourage the child to use executive skills already within her behavioral repertoire. Some parents resort to punishment or imposing penalties, but we generally prefer a more balanced approach with as much emphasis on the positive as possible. A critical shortcoming of a punishment approach is that it doesn't tell children what to do—it only tells them what *not* to do. Furthermore, this approach, which focuses on the negative, can damage the relationship between parents and children. All too often, parents who have taken a punitive approach say to us, "I don't have anything else to take away," and the child says, "I've got nothing to lose."

Reinforcing Executive Skills with Praise

As in the first scenario above, this may be as simple as providing praise and recognition. Parents might say to their 5-year-old, for instance, "You remembered to brush your teeth after breakfast without my having to remind you. That's great!" If you're inclined to believe virtue should be its own reward, remember that we're dealing with kids here. They're always seeking your approval, and getting it definitely encourages them to repeat the behavior so you'll repeat the praise. (Besides, what adult do you know who doesn't need praise at least sometimes?)

We've found, in fact, that praise is one of the most underappreciated (and underused) tools for promoting behavior change that parents have at their disposal. Skilled behavior specialists generally recommend that for every corrective statement directed at a child, parents make three positive statements. In practice this is a difficult ratio to reach. Still, it's a goal worth working toward.

We should also point out that some kinds of praise are more effective than others. Global praise ("Good girl!" "Great job!") is generally far less effective than more specific praise that is individualized to the child and to the behavior being reinforced. The box below outlines how praise can be delivered most effectively.

Effective Praise . . .

1. Is delivered immediately after the positive behavior occurs.
2. Specifies the particulars of the accomplishment ("Thank you for picking up your toys right away after I asked you").
3. Provides information to the child about the value of the accomplishment ("When you get ready for school quickly, it makes the morning go so smoothly!").
4. Lets the child know that he or she worked hard to accomplish the task ("I saw you really trying to control your temper!").
5. Orients the child to better appreciate her own task-related behavior and think about problem solving ("I like the way you thought about that and figured out a good solution to the problem").

Something Fun at the Finish Line

After praise, the next easiest motivator is to give the child something to look forward to after using the desired skill or completing the desired skill sequence. This is a well-worn strategy that most parents use to good effect to get children to do chores or other tasks that kids don't want to do. We've found over years of working with families (as well as being astute observers of our own behavior) that having something to look forward to when an aversive task is completed has an energizing effect. In more technical terms, it *kindles a positive drive state* that helps combat any negative thoughts or feelings we might have about the task in front of us. This approach can be effective with adults as well as children, and even small rewards can give us a boost. I (this is Peg talking) often reward myself with a game or two of *Free Cell* after finishing a difficult section of a psychological report I'm writing. And when I have a chore to do in the evening that feels like it requires a lot of effort (like making phone calls—something I hate to do), I allow myself to eat dessert only after I've finished the task.

Wording Incentives as Positives Rather Than Negatives

Children are often told, "You can't play video games until you pick up your bedroom" or "You can't go outside until you've loaded the dishwasher." We strongly recommend you turn it around to emphasize the positive: "As soon as you pick up your bedroom, you can play video games" or "You can go outside as soon as the dishwasher is loaded." The difference may seem subtle, but we believe it's important. When you stress access to a desired activity rather than lack of access to a desired activity, you're keeping your child's eyes on the prize and not the work that has to be done to get it. The behavioral data we've collected show that this shift really is effective: we've seen increases in direction following and decreases in task refusal and power struggles when adults use positive statements with kids rather than negative ones.

Using More Formal Incentive Systems

Praise and having something to look forward to are not always enough to motivate children to use difficult skills, however. In this case, you may find it helpful to use a more formal incentive system. If your child has ADHD, you may already be familiar with this kind of incentive system. If not, follow these steps:

Step 1: Describe the Problem Behavior and Set a Goal

This may sound familiar because it's identical to the first two steps listed in the previous chapter on teaching executive skills. As you may remember, it's important to describe the problem and goal behaviors as specifically as possible. For example, if forgetting to do chores after school is the problem, the goal might be "Joe will complete daily chores without reminders before 4:30 in the afternoon."

Step 2: Decide on Possible Rewards and Contingencies

The first step in designing a system of rewards and contingencies is to build a schedule so that less preferred tasks always precede more preferred tasks. This is another way of describing Grandma's law, which we told you about in Chapter 5. In some cases, this is all that's needed. When something more is necessary, incentive systems work best when children have a "menu" of rewards to choose from. One of the best ways to create this is to set up a system in which points can be earned for the goal behaviors and traded in for the reward the child wants to earn. The bigger the reward, the more points the child will need to earn it. The menu should include larger, more expensive rewards that may take a week or a month to earn and smaller, inexpensive rewards that can be earned daily. Rewards can include "material" reinforcers (such as favorite foods or small toys) as well as activity rewards (such as the chance to play a game with a parent, teacher, or friend). It may also be necessary to build contingencies into the system—usually access to a privilege after a task is done (such as the chance to watch a favorite TV show or the chance to talk on the telephone to a friend). An example of how this process might be applied to the problem of completing chores is in the box below.

While this book is directed primarily at things you can do at home, one effective way to use motivational strategies to improve executive skills at school is to link performance of the goal behavior at school with a reward at home. This is effective for a number of reasons. First of all, it provides a nice vehicle for home and school to work together to tackle a problem. Second, it serves as a mechanism for positive communication between home and school. And finally, parents often have available a wider array of reinforcers than are available to teachers. When a coordinated approach is used, a home–school report card is often the vehicle by which teachers communicate to parents how many points the child has earned that day.

Sample Incentive Planning Sheet

Problem behavior

Forgetting to do chores after school

Goal

Complete chores by 4:30 P.M. without reminders

Possible rewards (child earns 2 points for each day goal is met)

Daily (1 point)	Weekly (5 points)	Long-Term
Extra TV show	Chance to rent video game	Buy video game (20 points)
Extra video game time	Have friend spend night on weekend	Buy CD (12 points)

| Play game with Dad | Mom will make favorite dessert | Eat out (15 points) |
| Extra half-hour before bed | Chance to choose dinner menu | |

Possible Contingencies/Penalties

Can play with friends after school as soon as chores are done

Access to TV/video games after chores are done

Step 3: Write a Behavior Contract

The contract should say exactly what the child agrees to do and exactly what the parents' role and responsibilities will be. Along with points and rewards, be sure to praise your child for following the contract. Also be sure the contract is one you can live with. Avoid penalties you are either unable or unwilling to impose (for instance, if both parents work and are not at home, you won't be able to monitor whether your child is beginning his homework right after school, so an alternative contract may need to be written). A behavior contract to accompany the incentive system is depicted in the box shown on pages 117–118. Blank forms that you can use to design incentive systems and write behavior contracts are included at the end of this chapter.

Sample Behavior Contract

Child agrees to: complete chores by 4:30 P.M. without verbal reminders.

To help child reach goal, parents will: place a chore list on kitchen table before child comes home from school.

Child will earn: five points for each day he completes chores without verbal reminders. Points can be traded in for items on the reward menu.

If child fails to meet agreement, child will: not earn any points.

Step 4: Evaluate the Process and Make Changes If Necessary

We have to warn you that in our experience it's the rare incentive system that works perfectly the first time around. For one thing, kids are amazingly adept at figuring out the loopholes in any behavior contract ("You said I only had to *finish* my homework by 5:30—you didn't say anything about the work being done *right!*"). But in general it's common to have to tinker with the rules of the contract, the points allotted, or the specific rewards chosen before the contract works the way you want it to.

Parents often ask how they can develop this kind of system for one child in the family and not for all children because it may seem to be "rewarding" children with problems while neglecting those without. We have found that most siblings are understanding of this process if it's explained to them carefully. If there are problems, however, you have several choices:

1. Set up a similar system for other children with appropriate goals (*every* child has *something* he or she could be working to improve).
2. Make a more informal arrangement by promising to do something special from time to time with the other children in the family so they don't feel left out.
3. Have the child earn rewards that benefit the whole family (such as eating out at a Chinese restaurant).

Using Motivational Strategies to Reinforce Executive Skills in General

All the examples we've given you focus on a specific target behavior to be improved (remembering to do chores, earning good grades, picking up toys, etc.). You can use the same strategies to focus on helping your child develop executive skills more broadly rather than addressing single behaviors. If you decide you want to work on task initiation—for instance, every time your child starts a task without the need for reminders—you can reinforce the child for that. "Thanks for emptying the dishwasher right after you came home from school" and "I like the way you started your homework at 5 o'clock, just as we agreed on" are examples of specific praise that focuses on task initiation. If you feel you need to use a more powerful reinforcer, then each time your child starts something right away, or at the time agreed on, or without the need for more than one reminder, you can put a token in a jar. When the jar is full (or the child has earned the agreed-upon number of tokens), the reward is earned.

If you've stuck with us to this point, you should now have an understanding of the three broad approaches to managing your child's executive skill weaknesses. In the next section we move from "big picture" to practical applications. So if you're not yet sure how to use what you've learned so far, keep reading. We will give you teaching routines and vignettes drawn from our experience as parents and clinicians that solve the array of problems that arise in daily living because children have less-than-perfect executive skills.

INCENTIVE PLANNING SHEET

Problem Behavior

_____

_____

_____

_____

_____

Goal

_____

_____

_____

_____

_____

Possible Rewards

Daily	Weekly	Long-Term

Possible Contingencies/Penalties

_____

_____

_____

_____

_____

BEHAVIOR CONTRACT

Child agrees to: _____

_____

_____

_____

To help child reach goal, parents will: _____

_____

_____

_____

Child will earn: _____

_____

_____

_____

If child fails to meet agreement, child will: _____

_____

_____

_____

Part III

PUTTING IT ALL TOGETHER

9

....

Advance Organizer

In Chapters 6–8 you learned the ABCs of designing interventions to improve your child's executive skills: change the Antecedent (modify the environment), address the Behavior directly (teach the skill), and change the Consequence (provide incentives). Pretty straightforward, but where do you begin? How much are you really going to have to do to make a significant difference in your child's life?

As we've been promising since the beginning of this book, we're going to make the process of improving your child's executive skills easy by offering several approaches. How much you actively do will be your choice. You'll be able to have a measurable impact on your son or daughter within the bounds of your available time and energy.

We are, in fact, so thoroughly committed to making this process easy that the first and most important rule of thumb we want to offer is this:

1. First, Do the Minimum Necessary for Your Child to Be Successful

Sure, you can use everything we've explained in Chapters 5–8 and combine all the possible approaches to intervention from Chapters 9–21 to devise an elaborate, multicomponent plan. Eventually you may decide to do that. But you're reading this book to make your life easier at the same time as you're giving your child a boost toward the skills needed to be successful. So try the minimum intervention first:

• *If you can get away with simple environmental modifications that your child will eventually internalize on her own, by all means do it.* A note on the kitchen table that says *Please walk the dog as soon as you get home from school* is an example of an environmental modification. If you leave the note for 3 weeks, and then don't leave it, does your child still remember to walk the dog? If so, then her own working memory is kicking in. If you ask your child to estimate how long it will take him to do his math homework and you compare his estimates to the actual time and see that he's becoming more accurate, then you know he is refining his time management skills. (See Chapter 6 for a detailed discussion of how to modify the environment to enhance executive skill development.)

• *Or if you think your child already has a particular skill but needs to be encouraged to use it, a motivational strategy alone may be sufficient.* Maybe you've set up a folder system to help your daughter keep track of homework assignments, but she keeps stuffing the work into random books and notebooks. A motivational strategy might look like this: By showing you her folders when she finishes her homework each night she can earn 5 points. When she has 25 points, she can download a song from the iTunes store for her iPod. Or maybe your son needs to be helped to learn not to say mean things to his little brother. A motivational strategy for this situation might be this: Target the hour before dinner and place a token in a jar for every 10 minutes that you hear him say nothing mean. If he's earned 4 tokens by dinner, he gets his favorite dessert. (See Chapter 8 for further instructions for how to set up motivational systems.)

• *If you believe your child might benefit substantially just from some scaffolding and game playing, give that a shot first.* Learning how to win and lose gracefully (that is, develop emotional control) is particularly well suited to game playing. Ditto learning to wait your turn or tolerate a teammate's weaker skill level (see Chapter 7).

Chances are, though, that there will be some skills that need to be taught and some skills that require a multipronged approach. Take, for example, long-term school assignments. Breaking down an assignment into subtasks and timelines is something that many kids simply need to be taught to do. Being taught the process (as we lay it out in Chapter 10) and then being walked through it a few times for practice may be all they need to acquire these skills. Or consider the skill of time management. If your child can't manage time because she doesn't know how long it takes to do certain tasks, you can teach her time estimation skills and then build in some practice, and that may be all she'll need to become skilled at time management. Chapters 9–21 will show you how to teach each of the 11 executive skills when the problem is that the child just doesn't know how.

But what if you teach a skill, get your child to practice it, and the child still pulls a disappearing act or resorts to a variety of stall tactics whenever certain tasks come up? This is a sure sign that you need a multipronged approach. Sometimes just understanding how the process works isn't enough, and the child finds particular skills demand so much effort from him that he'll do anything to avoid the tasks involving them. For those cases, Chapters 9–21 also illustrate how you can put together a program that incorporates motivational techniques and troubleshooting so that even the tasks that seem "impossible" to your child right now eventually become manageable.

Here's what you'll do when you need to take a more targeted approach to giving your child a skill he lacks:

2. Next, Learn the Principles That Underlie Effective Strategies

This chapter offers guidelines for intervening in lagging executive skills. The principles you'll read here form the foundation for all the strategies you'll learn to use in this book. Read this chapter before you start using any intervention with your child. Come back to it when a strategy you're trying isn't working; it may be because you've forgotten an important guideline and need to tweak the strategy to integrate it.

3. Now Tackle Specific Daily Routines

In our work, parents bring up a certain predictable set of daily problems associated with executive skill weaknesses over and over. Parents of preschoolers and early elementary school-aged children often complain about their child's inability to get through a morning routine, get ready for bed efficiently, clean up bedrooms or playrooms, or control their temper. Parents of children in upper elementary school and middle school often complain about their kids' failure to get their homework done, keep their notebooks organized, or carry out long-term projects. We know that battles over these regular routines can ruin your day and your child's—day after day and week after week. You can all get pretty quick relief by attacking these routines directly with the instructional schemes we've created for you. *That's why we strongly recommend that you try using the ready-made interventions in Chapter 10 as your next step after you've tried the minimal help listed above.* Chapter 10 gives you detailed plans, including any forms or checklists you need to implement the plan, for 20 different daily routines that often cause problems for kids with weak executive skills.

Choosing a Routine to Tackle First

You'll find it easy to dive in if you look through the list of routines at the beginning of the chapter and immediately zero in on one that feels like the bane of your existence. Maybe the battle over getting ready for school leaves your child too upset to concentrate during the first couple hours of school, and as a result his reading grades are taking a nosedive. Or trying to wrestle your child into bed at night leaves you so worked up that you rarely get a good night's sleep. In cases like these you know which routine to tackle first.

But what if you look through the list of daily routines and can point to a dozen of them that cause you and your child trouble every day? How do you know where to start? Here are a few ideas:

• *Start with the problem that, if that one thing cleared up, your child's life—and yours!—would go so much more smoothly.* Because improved quality of life is one of our bottom lines, this is often the best place to start. Maggie wasn't sure that it mattered that much to 6-year-old Cindy's well-being that bedtime felt like one wrestling match (in fact, in her worst moments she was sure Cindy thoroughly enjoyed this battle of wills). But it left Maggie exhausted, unable to fall asleep herself, and feeling like an incompetent parent who missed the cuddling during bedtime stories when her little girl was 4. So she chose bedtime as the routine to tackle first.

• *Start with a problem that is small and can be tackled easily.* The benefit of this approach is that you can achieve some quick success and build your confidence to try something a little more challenging. Brad chose helping his son Trey do the chore of feeding the dogs every night. It was a simple chore that took very little time, but Trey never seemed to remember to do it and then drove his father crazy responding with "Just a minute!" numerous times when reminded. You too can break down a routine we've laid out to make it even simpler by targeting a very simple chore to address.

• *Give your child a choice of what to tackle first.* This appeals to us, too, because this increases the child's ownership of the problem and the solution—and it taps the child's need for mastery and control. Jessie decided she wanted help with practicing the piano. Her grandparents were coming to town for her recital, and her desire to perform well for them served as a built-in incentive.

• *Choose one where the implementation can be shared.* If you and your spouse agree on the target problem and you can share the burden for solving it, the effort required of you alone is lessened, which makes it more likely that the intervention will work. Read through the routine and decide who will do what when. Make sure you agree on the details, since, as we all know, the devil is in the details. For the Gonzaleses, homework was perfect. One parent would help their son with getting his math done while the other cooked dinner, then the cook would help him stick to his reading assignment while the other parent did the dishes.

• *Think about long-term goals.* This is especially important with older children, where adulthood is beginning to appear on the horizon. When I realized that my then 13-year-old son (this is Peg talking) had some significant executive skill problems in a number of domains, I wasn't sure what to focus on. I finally asked myself, *What skills will be absolutely critical, for both success in college and success on the job?* With that in mind, I decided a clean bedroom was a low priority, while meeting deadlines and remembering everything he had to get done were high priorities. Once I'd made that decision, I began monitoring his homework by asking him two questions when he came home from school every day: *What do you have to do? When are you going to do it?*

Which Executive Skills Will You Be Building in Your Child?

Each routine covered in Chapter 10 lists up front the executive skills that the routine demands. You'll notice that all of these routines, while designed to address one particular problem in daily life, actually aim at working on a number of executive skills simultaneously. Kids who have trouble getting through a morning routine, for instance, often struggle with task initiation (they're slow to get started), sustained attention (they have trouble persisting long enough to get it done), and working memory (they lose track of what they're supposed to be doing). By putting in place an intervention to deal with one problem, then, you're actually working to improve several executive skills simultaneously. You can probably guess that in time this means you may see improvements in other routines involving the same executive skills without directly intervening in those routines. (As we've noted, though, don't expect this to happen overnight or even this month. Sometimes, for some kids, you'll have to keep the aids in place for quite a while before the skills are internalized.)

4. Finally, Target Specific Executive Skill Weaknesses

If your child's problems are pretty pervasive, especially if Chapter 2 helped you identify just one or two executive skill weaknesses behind all the trouble, or the routines that cause the greatest problems aren't covered in Chapter 10, you'll want to go beyond following our instructions and design your own strategies. Some of you may want to use the ready-made routines in Chapter 10 *and* design your own plans. Each of Chapters 11–21 goes into depth on a particular skill, giving you additional information on it, helping you look more closely at your child's deficits in the skill, and then showing you how other parents have devised effective interventions. You can pick any problem that your child struggles with and design a plan of attack that will either teach the skill discussed in that chapter or help the child practice and enhance the skill when the child has it but doesn't use it well. Each of Chapters 11–21 also gives some general tips for strengthening the skill outside of a fully drawn intervention scheme.

How Do You Decide Which Executive Skills to Target?

If you start by using the plans we've created for Chapter 10, you'll probably notice that the routines your child needs help with most all entail the same executive skills. This is one way to determine which individual skills to work further on. You also have the questionnaires (pp. 34–43) that you used to assess your child's executive skills in Chapter 2 to go on. Finally, you can confirm your initial assessment of your child by filling in the brief questionnaire at the beginning of each of the skills chapters that discusses the skill you believe your child lacks.

These questionnaires are similar to the scale you completed in Chapter 2, but this time we ask you to rate how well or how often you feel your child exhibits each of the behaviors listed so you'll know whether all you need is the general tips or whether you should design your own full-blown intervention strategies. If you decide to craft your own intervention, you can draw from all the ideas in Chapters

5–8. Because we're such strong believers in checklists, we've put one together to help you remember all the elements you need to at least consider when creating a plan to help your child cope with his or her particular problem or particular executive skill weakness. It is shown on page 127. In case you need a refresher about the meaning of any of the items on the checklist, we've noted where in the book the item is discussed.

Tips for Success in Designing Your Own Program

Whether you use our interventions from Chapter 10 or design your own—or both—your plan is more likely to succeed if you keep these ideas in mind:

- *Help your child own the plan.* Involve your child as much as possible in designing the intervention. Listen to her input, incorporate her suggestions, and honor her requests whenever possible. Be willing to compromise to increase your child's ownership of the plan. Remember, as we discussed in Chapter 5, one of the forces that shape children's behavior is a drive for mastery and control—use this to your advantage whenever you can.

- *Remember the importance of goodness of fit.* Keep in mind that what you think would work for you may not be a good fit for your child. We've found, in particular, that organizational schemes that work for one individual have no appeal to another. Ask your child what will work for him.

- *Take opportunities to brainstorm with your child.* Brainstorming itself builds executive skills. If your son can't think of anything that might work for him, turn it into a brainstorming session or offer him choices and see which one feels right to him.

- *Expect to have to tweak your strategies.* Assume that the first plan you design will need to be adjusted. In Chapter 10, we list some modifications and adjustments you may want to consider. In the skills chapters (Chapters 11–21), many of the scenarios we present show how the initial attempts met with some success but also needed to be tinkered with to produce the maximum benefit.

- *Whenever possible, practice, role-play, or rehearse the procedure before putting it in place.* This will be particularly important if the target executive skill is response inhibition or emotional control. Because things can happen quickly in real life and because the problem behavior often occurs in emotionally charged situations, the more practice the child can get when her emotions are not at their peak, the more likely she'll be able to follow the script in the heat of the moment.

- *Always use lots of praise and positive feedback.* Even if you're using other incentives, you shouldn't drop the praise. Because the goal with any incentive program is to fade the need for tangible rewards, social reinforcers (praise and positive feedback) help the child transition away from the tangible reward.

- *Use visual reminders whenever possible.* All too often, verbal reminders "go in

DESIGNING INTERVENTIONS

Intervention steps	Reference page(s)
1. Establish behavioral goal. 　Problem behavior: _____ 　Goal behavior: _____	99 99–100
2. What environmental supports will be provided? (Check all that apply.) 　___ Change physical or social environment (e.g., add physical barriers, reduce distractions, provide organizational structures, reduce social complexity) 　___ Change the nature of the task (e.g., shorten it, build in breaks, give something to look forward to, create a schedule, build in choice, make the task more fun) 　___ Change the way adults interact with the child (e.g., rehearsal, prompts, reminders, coaching, praise, debriefing, feedback)	83–85 85–87 87–91
3. What procedure will be followed to teach the skill? Who will teach the skill/supervise the procedure?_____ _____ What steps will the child follow? 　1. _____ 　2. _____ 　3. _____ 　4. _____ 　5. _____ 　6. _____	101–107
4. What incentives will be used to encourage the child to learn, practice, or use the skill? (Check all that apply.) 　___ Specific praise 　___ Something to look forward to when the task (or a piece of the task) is done 　___ A menu of rewards and penalties Daily reward possibilities: _____ _____ _____ Weekly reward possibilities: _____ _____ _____ Long-term reward possibilities: _____ _____ _____	110–118 112 114–117

one ear and out the other." When you do use verbal cues, use them to refer your child to visuals such as picture schedules, lists, checklists, written mottos, or slogans: "Check your list." "What comes next on your schedule?"

• *Start small(er)!* Begin with a behavior that's a minor annoyance and build in lots of success up front so that you and your child experience success right away. When you move on to bigger problems, still plan for success by making the initial goals attainable. Your long-term goal may be to get your son to do all his homework independently without needing your presence, but a reasonable first step might be to get him to work by himself for 2 minutes. If you know you tend to overreach, take your first idea for a goal and cut it in half (half the time, half the work, half the challenge, half the improvement).

• *Whenever possible, measure progress by finding something to count, then graph the results.* If you're not sure whether the program is working, figure out a way to collect data to answer the question. Graphs, by the way, can be incredibly reinforcing to children (actually, to people of all ages). If you're using point systems, you have the feedback mechanism built in, but we recommend turning the points into a graph, too. Some examples of behaviors that can be counted and graphed are: missing homework assignments per week; number of "meltdowns" per day; number of school days per week that the child remembered everything he had to bring to and from school; number of times an unexpected change of plans was handled without crying; number of evenings per week that homework was finished before the agreed-upon time.

What If Your Child Wants No Part of Your Plans?

If, after reading through the teaching routines, scenarios, and behavior plans, you're all gung-ho to try something but your child wants no part of it, here are some things to try:

• *Try negotiating.* Be willing to give up something to get something in return (but make sure both sides win).

• *Consider more powerful reinforcers.* We've found that parents and teachers often err on the side of stinginess. Remember that what we're often asking children with executive skill deficits to do is tasks that require huge efforts from them. If the task looks bigger to them than the reward, they'll continue to resist the task.

• *If your child resists all your attempts to engage him in developing a behavior plan (this is most likely to occur in adolescence), you can still build in logical or natural consequences.* To get to the privileges your child wants, arrange it so she has to go through you ("I'll be happy to take you to the mall so you can hang out with your friends, but first you need to clean your bedroom").

• *If nothing seems to work, and the problems are severe enough, seek outside help such as a therapist, coach, or tutor.* Chapter 22 offers suggestions for how to do this.

The Game Plan at a Glance

1. First try modifying the environment (Chapter 6), using scaffolding and games (Chapter 7), or providing incentives.
2. If that's not enough, learn the principles and guidelines behind effective strategies for building executive skills (Chapter 9).
3. Start intervening by using our ready-made plans to tackle especially problematic daily routines (Chapter 10).
4. If that's not enough, work on specific executive skills (Chapters 11–21).
   - Follow general tips for helping the child use weak skills more effectively and consistently.
   - If the child lacks the skill altogether, design your own interventions, following the "Designing Interventions" framework (this chapter).

10

Ready-Made Plans for Teaching Your Child to Complete Daily Routines

The following 20 routines are the ones that children tend to struggle with most. We've grouped them starting with home routines, then those related to school, with the tasks requiring emotional control, flexibility, and response inhibition at the end. Glance through the list and you'll undoubtedly zero right in on the areas where you and your child need help. Refer back to Chapter 9 if you identify several and don't know where to start. We've given the chapter number for each executive skill the routine addresses if you decide you want to do more targeted work on specific skills.

Adapting the Interventions for Your Child's Age

In some cases, the ages for which the interventions are appropriate will be dictated by the developmental task involved in the routine or by the school curriculum. We don't expect first graders to study for tests (except spelling tests), to do long-term projects, or to write papers, so these routines were not designed for that age group. Other routines may be applicable for a range of ages. Because many of the routines were written for children in the middle of the age range covered by this book (mid-elementary school), here are some suggestions for how to adjust the strategies for younger and older children where that seems appropriate.

General guidelines for developing instructional routines for young children:

- Keep them short.
- Reduce the number of steps involved.
- Use pictures as cues rather than written lists or written instructions.
- Be prepared to provide cues and supervision, and in some cases you'll need to help the child follow the routine, working side by side.

General guidelines for developing instructional routines for older children:

- Make them full partners in the design of the routine, the selection of rewards, and the troubleshooting that may be required to improve the routine.
- Be willing to negotiate rather than dictate.
- Whenever possible, use visual cues rather than verbal cues (because these sound a lot like nagging to an older child).

1. Getting Ready in the Morning

Executive skills addressed: Task initiation (Chapter 15), sustained attention (Chapter 14), working memory (Chapter 12).

Ages: Specifics we've included are for ages 7–10, but this routine is very easy to customize for younger and older children just by changing the sophistication of the tasks.

1. Sit down with your child and together make a list of the things to be done before leaving for school in the morning (or just starting the day for younger kids).
2. Decide together the order in which the tasks should be done.
3. Turn the list into a checklist. (The checklists that follow are just samples; you can use them as is or just as a model, with your own tasks listed in the left column.)
4. Make multiple copies and attach them to a clipboard.
5. Talk through with your child how the process will work from the moment the child wakes up. Explain that in the beginning you will cue your child to do each item on the list and that he or she will check off each item as it is completed.
6. Rehearse or role-play the process so that your child understands how it will work—that is, walk through each step, with the child pretending to do each step and check it off.
7. Determine what time the whole routine should be finished in order to get to school on time (or in order to have some time to play before going to school or to get to whatever the child needs to do).
8. Put the system to work. Initially you should cue your child to begin the first step, watch as he or she does the step, prompt to check off the step on the checklist, praise the child for completing each step, and cue your child to do the next step. Continue the process with supervision until the entire routine is completed.
9. Once the child has internalized the process and is able to complete the routine independently within time constraints, the checklist can be faded.

Fading the Supervision

1. Cue your child to begin and supervise throughout the routine, providing frequent praise and encouragement as well as constructive feedback.
2. Cue your child to begin, make sure he or she starts each step, and then go away and come back for the next step.
3. Cue your child to begin, check on him or her intermittently (every two steps, then every three steps, etc.).
4. Cue your child to begin and have him or her check in with you at the end.

Modifications/Adjustments

1. If necessary, add a reinforcer for completing the process on time or with minimal reminders. Or give the child a point for each step in the process completed with minimal reminders (agree on how many reminders will be permissible for the child to earn the point).
2. Set a kitchen timer—or have the child set the timer—at the beginning of each step and challenge the child to complete the step before the timer rings.
3. Adjust the time or the schedule as needed—for example, wake the child up earlier or see if there are any items on the list that can be dropped or done the night before.
4. Rather than making a checklist, write each task on a separate index card and have the child hand in the card and get a new one as each step is completed.
5. For younger children, use pictures rather than words, keep the list short, and assume that you'll need to continue to cue the child.
6. The same approach can be adapted for children who need help specifically with making sure they're taking everything to school that they need. A sample checklist for this is also provided.

MORNING ROUTINE CHECKLIST

Task	Number of reminders Tally marks (////)	Done (✓)
Get up		
Get dressed		
Eat breakfast		
Put dishes in dishwasher		
Brush teeth		
Brush hair		
Get backpack ready for school		

GETTING READY FOR SCHOOL CHECKLIST

Task	Done (✓)
ALL homework completed	
ALL homework in appropriate place (notebook, folder, etc.)	

Items to go to school	Placed in backpack (✓)
Homework	
Notebooks/folders	
Textbooks	
Silent reading book	
Permission slips	
Lunch money	
Sports/P.E. clothes/equipment	
Notes for teacher	
Assignment book	
Other:	
Other:	

2. Bedroom Cleaning

Executive skills addressed: Task initiation (Chapter 15), sustained attention (Chapter 14), working memory (Chapter 12), organization (Chapter 17).

Ages: Specifics we've included are for ages 7–10, but this routine is very easy to customize for younger and older children just by changing the sophistication of the tasks.

1. Sit down with your child and together make a list of the steps involved in cleaning his or her bedroom. They might look like this:

   - Put dirty clothes in laundry
   - Put clean clothes in dresser/closet
   - Put toys away on toy shelves or in boxes/bins
   - Put books on bookshelves
   - Clean off desk surface
   - Throw away trash
   - Return things to other rooms (dirty dishes to kitchen, towels to bathroom, etc.)

2. Turn the list into a checklist (a sample based on the list above follows; use it as is or as a model with your own tasks in the left column).
3. Decide when the chore will be done.
4. Decide what kinds of cues and reminders the child will get before and during the task.
5. Decide how much help the child will get in the beginning (the long-term goal should be for the child to clean the room alone).
6. Decide how the quality of the task will be judged.
7. Put the routine in place with the agreed-upon cues, reminders, and help.

Fading the Supervision

1. Cue your child to begin and supervise throughout the routine, providing frequent praise and encouragement as well as constructive feedback.
2. Cue your child to begin, make sure he or she starts each step, and then go away and come back for the next step.
3. Cue your child to begin, then check on him or her intermittently (every two steps, then every three steps, etc.).
4. Cue your child to begin and have him or her check in with you at the end.

Modifications/Adjustments

1. Add a reinforcer if needed. This could either be giving the child something to look forward to doing when the chore is completed, or giving the child points for completing each step, with rewards selected from a reward menu. Rewarding your child for completing each step with no more than one or two reminders or prompts is another way to organize a reward system.
2. If even with your constant presence, cueing, and praise, the child can't follow the routine, begin by working alongside your child, sharing each task.
3. If even that is too much, consider using a backward chaining approach—you clean the entire room except for one small piece and have the child do that piece with supervision and praise. Gradually add in more pieces for the child to do until the child is doing the entire job.
4. Make the room easier to clean—use storage bins that the child can "dump" toys into and label each bin.
5. Take a photograph of what a "clean room" looks like, so when your child completes the task, you can ask him or her to rate his or her performance by comparing his or her work to the photo.
6. For younger children, use pictures of each step rather than words; reduce the number of steps; assume the child will need help rather than expecting him or her to work alone.

BEDROOM-CLEANING CHECKLIST

Task	Number of reminders Tally marks (////)	Done (✓)
Put dirty clothes in laundry		
Put clean clothes in dresser/closet		
Put toys away (toy shelves, toy box)		
Put books on bookshelves		
Tidy desk		
Throw away trash		
Return things to other rooms (e.g., dishes, cups, towels, sports stuff)		
Other:		
Other:		

3. Putting Belongings Away

Executive skills addressed: Organization (Chapter 17), task initiation (Chapter 15), sustained attention (Chapter 14), working memory (Chapter 12).

Ages: Specifics we've included are for ages 7–10, but this routine is very easy to customize for younger and older children just by changing the list of belongings.

1. With your child, make a list of the items your child routinely leaves out of place around the house.
2. Identify the proper location for each item.
3. Decide when the item will be put away (for example, as soon as I get home from school, after I finish my homework, just before bed, right after I finish using it, etc.).
4. Decide on a "rule" for reminders—how many reminders are allowed before a penalty is imposed (for example, the belonging is placed off limits, or another privilege is withdrawn). A sample checklist follows.
5. Decide where the checklist will be kept.

Fading the Supervision

1. Remind your child that you're working on learning to put things away where they belong.
2. Put the checklist in a prominent place and remind your child to use it each time he or she puts something away.
3. Praise or thank your child each time he or she puts something away.
4. After your child has followed the system for a couple of weeks, with lots of praise and reminders from you, fade the reminders. Keep the checklist in a prominent place, but now you may want to impose a penalty for forgetting. For example, if a toy or a desired object or article of clothing is not put away, your child may lose access to it for a period of time. If it's an object that can't be taken away (as in a school backpack), then impose a fine or withdraw a privilege.

Modifications/Adjustments

1. Add an incentive if needed. One way to do this would be to place a set number of tokens in a jar each day and withdraw one token each time the child fails to put away an item on time. Tokens can be traded in for small tangible or activity rewards.
2. If remembering to put items away right after use or at different times during the day is too difficult, arrange for a daily pick-up time when all belongings need to be returned to their appropriate locations.
3. For younger children, use pictures, keep the list short, and assume the child will need cues and/or help for a longer period of time.

PUTTING BELONGINGS AWAY

Belonging	Where does it go?	When will I put it away?	Reminders needed (///)	Done! (✓)
Sports equipment				
Outerwear (jackets, gloves, etc.)				
Other clothing				
Shoes				
Homework				
Backpack				
Other:				
Other:				

From *Smart but Scattered* by Peg Dawson and Richard Guare. Copyright 2009 by The Guilford Press.

4. Completing Chores

Executive skills addressed: Task initiation (Chapter 15), sustained attention (Chapter 14), working memory (Chapter 12).

Ages: Any age; even preschoolers can be assigned simple, short chores.

1. Sit down with your child and make a list of chores that need to be done.
2. Decide how long it will take to do each chore.
3. Decide when (day and/or time) the chore needs to be done.
4. Create a schedule so you and your child can keep track of the chore. A sample schedule follows.
5. Decide where the checklist will be kept.

Fading the Supervision

1. Cue your child to begin each chore and supervise throughout, providing frequent praise and encouragement as well as constructive feedback.
2. Cue your child to begin, make sure he or she starts each step, and then go away and come back for the next step.
3. Cue your child to begin, check on him or her intermittently (every two steps, then every three steps, etc.).
4. Cue your child to begin and have him or her check in with you at the end.

Modifications/Adjustments

1. If necessary, add a reinforcer for completing the process on time or with minimal reminders. Or give the child a point for each step in the process completed with minimal reminders (agree on how many reminders will be permissible for the child to earn the point).
2. Set a kitchen timer—or have the child set the timer—at the beginning of each step and challenge the child to complete the step before the timer rings.
3. Adjust the time or the schedule as needed—for example, wake the child up earlier or see if any items on the list can be dropped or done the night before.
4. Rather than making a checklist, write each task on a separate index card and have the child hand in the card and get a new one as each step is completed.
5. For younger children, use pictures rather than words, keep the chores very brief, don't give too many chores, and assume the child will need cues and/or help to complete the chore.

COMPLETING CHORES

Chore	How long will it take?	When will you do it? Day Time
1.		
2.		
3.		
4.		

	Sunday	Monday	Tuesday	Wednesday	Thursday	Friday	Saturday
	Chore done (✓)	Chore done (✓)	Chore done (✓)	Chore done (✓)	Chore done (✓)	Chore done (✓)	Chore done (✓)
1							
2							
3							
4							

5. Maintaining a Practice Schedule*

Executive skills addressed: Task initiation (Chapter 15), sustained attention (Chapter 14), planning (Chapter 16).

Ages: Mainly 8–14; for younger children, activities like dance, music, and sports should be designed more for fun than for skill acquisition, although younger kids do build skills during ballet lessons, soccer, tumbling classes, and the like.

1. Ideally, this process should begin when your child first decides on a skill he or she wants to develop that requires daily or consistent practice. Before you and he or she decide to go ahead with this, have a conversation about what will be required to master the skill (or to get good enough for it to be enjoyable!). Talk about how often he or she will need to practice, how long practice sessions will last, what other responsibilities he or she has, and whether there is enough time in the schedule to make consistent practice possible.
2. Create a weekly schedule for when the practice will take place. A sample follows.
3. Talk about what cues or reminders your child might need to remember to start the practice.
4. Talk about how you and your child will decide whether the process is working. In other words, what are the criteria for success to signal that your child should continue?
5. Decide how long you will keep at it before deciding whether to continue. Many parents have strong feelings that when a child decides to take up something like a musical instrument or a sport (especially if money is involved, such as buying an expensive instrument), he or she should "sign on" for enough time to make the expense and commitment worth it. Given that many children tire of these kinds of activities within a relatively short period of time, it makes sense to come to some agreement in advance for the minimum amount of time you expect your child to stick with it before you can discuss giving it up.

Fading the Supervision

1. Cue your child to begin the practice at the agreed-on time and to check off on the checklist when he or she has finished. Place the checklist in a prominent place so that it alone can eventually act as the cue.
2. Use a written reminder and the checklist. If your child doesn't begin within 5 minutes of the agreed-on time, provide a verbal reminder. If he or she *does* begin on time, provide positive reinforcement for this.

---

*For a musical instrument, sport, or other skill that requires consistent practice.

Modifications/Adjustments

1. You and your child may want to pick a start time that's easy to remember—such as right after dinner or right after a favorite daily TV program. This way, the previous activity actually serves as a cue to begin the next activity.
2. If your child is having trouble remembering to start the practice without reminders, have him or her set a kitchen timer or an alarm clock (or a watch alarm) as a reminder.
3. If your child resists practicing as much as you originally agreed on, consider changing the schedule rather than giving up. Make the practice sessions shorter, schedule them for fewer days, break them in two with a brief break between them, or give them something to look forward to when the practice is finished (for example, schedule the practices *just before* a preferred activity).
4. If you find yourself thinking you need to add a reinforcer to make the practices more attractive to your child, it may be time to rethink the whole process. If your child is reluctant to practice as much as is needed to acquire the skill, this is a signal that he or she may not care so much about learning the skill after all. Many times it is parents who want children to learn something (particularly a musical instrument) and the process is not being driven by the child at all. If this is the case, be up front about it with your child—and then add the reinforcer to persuade your child to work on the skill.

LEARNING A NEW SKILL

BEFORE you begin, answer the following questions:

1. What do I want to learn?

2. Why do I want to learn this?

3. What will be involved in learning the skill (lessons, practice, etc.) and how much time will be involved?

What needs to be done	When will this happen?	How much time will it take?
Lessons		
Practice		
Other (e.g., games, exhibitions, recitals)		

4. Will I have to give up anything I'm doing now to fit this into my schedule?

If you decide you want to go ahead, plan your schedule by filling in the boxes that follow. Write what time each activity will take place and how long it will last. You can use this to keep track of your practices as well by crossing off each practice after you've finished it.

	Monday	Tuesday	Wednesday	Thursday	Friday	Saturday	Sunday
Lessons							
Practice							
Games, exhibitions, recitals							

6. Bedtime

Executive skills addressed: Task initiation (Chapter 15), sustained attention (Chapter 14), working memory (Chapter 12).

Ages: Specifics we've included are for ages 7–10, but this routine is very easy to customize for younger and older children just by changing the sophistication of the tasks.

1. Talk with your child about what time bedtime is. Make a list of all the things that need to be done before bedtime. This might include picking up toys, getting out clothes for the next day, making sure his or her backpack is ready for school (see Homework), putting on pajamas, brushing teeth, and washing face or bathing.
2. Turn the list into a checklist or picture schedule. A sample follows.
3. Talk about how long each task on the list will take. If you want, time each task with a stopwatch so you know exactly how long each task takes.
4. Add up the total amount of time and subtract that from the bedtime hour so you know when your child should begin the bedtime routine (for example, if bedtime is 8 o'clock and it will take a half hour to complete the routine, your child should start the routine at 7:30).
5. Prompt your child to begin the routine at the agreed-on time.
6. Supervise your child at each step, encouraging him or her to "check your list to see what's next" and providing praise for completion of each task.

Fading the Supervision

1. Cue your child to begin and supervise throughout the routine, providing frequent praise and encouragement as well as constructive feedback.
2. Cue your child to begin, make sure he or she starts each step, and then go away and come back for the next step.
3. Cue your child to begin, check on him or her intermittently (every two steps, then every three steps, etc.).
4. Cue your child to begin and have him or her check in with you at the end.

Modifications/Adjustments

1. Build in rewards or penalties. For instance, if your child completes the routine at or before the specified bedtime, he or she earns a little extra time before the lights have to go off. If he or she does not complete the routine by bedtime, the next night he or she has to begin the routine 15 minutes earlier.
2. Set the kitchen timer or give your child a stopwatch to use to help him or her keep track of how long each step is taking.
3. Rather than making a checklist, write each task on a separate index card and have the child hand in the card and get a new one as each step is completed.
4. For younger children, use pictures rather than words and assume the child will need cueing and/or supervision.

BEDTIME ROUTINE

Task	Number of reminders Tally marks (/ / / /)	Done (✓)
Pick up toys		
Make sure backpack is ready for school		
Make a list of anything you have to remember to do tomorrow		
Get clothes ready for next day		
Put on pajamas		
Wash face or bathe		
Brush teeth		

7. Desk Cleaning

Executive skills addressed: Task initiation (Chapter 15), sustained attention (Chapter 14), organization (Chapter 17), planning (Chapter 16).

Ages: Specifics we've included are for ages 7–10, but of course most 7-year-olds don't spend a lot of time at a desk, so if you need to customize for other ages, it will likely be for older children—just make the tasks more sophisticated.

First Steps: Cleaning the Desk

1. Take everything out of the desk.
2. Decide what items will go in which drawer. Make labels to put on the drawers.
3. Put appropriate items in the correct drawers.
4. Have a bin near the desk to hold paper that can be recycled.
5. Decide what items should go on top of the desk (a pencil holder, stapler, wire baskets for papers in current use and for things that need to be filed, etc.). Consider putting a bulletin board next to the desk to hold reminders as well as mementos.
6. Place items where your child wants them.
7. Take a picture of what the desk looks like to use as a model. Put the photo on the wall or bulletin board near the desk.

Steps for Maintaining a Clean Desk

1. Before beginning homework or any other desk project, make sure the desk looks like the photo. If not, put things away so the desk does look like the photo.
2. After finishing homework, put everything away so that the desk again looks like the photograph. This step could also be built into a bedtime routine.
3. Once a week, go through the baskets and decide what needs to stay in the basket, what can be filed, and what should be thrown away/recycled.

Fading the Supervision

1. Cue your child for each step in the maintenance procedure and supervise throughout the routine, providing frequent praise and encouragement as well as constructive feedback.
2. Cue your child to begin, make sure he or she starts step 1 of the procedure, and come back at the end to make sure he or she finished. Do the same with step 2. At step 3, stay with your child to assist in basket cleaning.
3. Cue your child for all three steps of the maintenance procedure but leave and check in at the end.
4. Remind your child to begin the procedure. At a later point (such as just before

bed), check in to make sure the desk is clean. Provide praise and constructive feedback.

Modifications/Adjustments

1. As your child follows the process, continue to refine it. For instance, there may be better ways of organizing things on top of the desk or in the drawers, and these changes should be incorporated into the process.
2. Visit an office supply store to see what kind of materials might help your child establish and maintain a system for keeping the desk uncluttered and materials readily available for use.
3. As with other procedures, build in a reinforcer for following the routine as necessary.

CLEAN DESK CHECKLIST							
Task	Monday	Tuesday	Wednesday	Thursday	Friday	Saturday	Sunday
Desk surface picked up							
Baskets cleared							
Desk matches photograph							

From *Smart but Scattered* by Peg Dawson and Richard Guare. Copyright 2009 by The Guilford Press.

8. Homework

Executive skills addressed: Task initiation (Chapter 15), sustained attention (Chapter 14), planning (Chapter 16), time management (Chapter 18), metacognition (Chapter 21).

Ages: 7–14.

1. Explain to your child that making a plan for homework is a good way to learn how to make plans and schedules. Explain that when he or she gets home from school, before doing anything else, he or she will make a homework plan using the form that you will provide (the form follows).
2. The steps the child should follow:
   a. Write down all assignments (this can be shorthand because more detailed directions should be in your child's agenda book or on worksheets).
   b. Make sure he or she has all the materials needed for each assignment.
   c. Determine whether he or she will need any help to complete the assignment and who will provide the help.
   d. Estimate how long each assignment will take.
   e. Write down when he or she will start each assignment.
   f. Show the plan to you so you can help make adjustments if needed (for example, with time estimations).
3. Cue your child to start homework at the time listed in the plan.
4. Monitor your child's performance throughout. Depending on the child, this may mean staying with him or her from start to finish, or it may mean checking up periodically.

Fading the Supervision

1. Cue your child to make the plan and to begin the routine, providing frequent praise and encouragement as well as constructive feedback. If necessary, sit with your child as he or she does the homework.
2. Cue your child to make the plan and to start homework on schedule. Check in frequently, providing praise and encouragement.
3. Cue your child to make the plan and start homework on schedule. Ask your child to check in with you when the homework is done.

Modifications/Adjustments

1. If your child resists writing the plan, you do the writing, but have your child tell you what to write.
2. If your child tends to forget assignments that may not be written down, modify

the planner to list every possible subject and talk about each subject with your child to jog his or her memory about assignments.

3. Create a separate calendar for long-term projects so that your child can keep track of the work that needs to be done on them (see Long-Term Projects).

4. Build in rewards for starting/ending homework on time or for remembering to do it without reminders.

5. For younger children, simply establishing a set time and place to do homework may be sufficient because they tend to have only one or two assignments per night. Asking them to estimate how long it will take to do each assignment may be useful because this helps train time management skills.

DAILY HOMEWORK PLANNER

Date:

Subject/assignment	Do I have all the materials?	Do I need help?	Who will help me?	How long will it take?	When will I start?	Done (✓)
	Yes ☐ No ☐	Yes ☐ No ☐				
	Yes ☐ No ☐	Yes ☐ No ☐				
	Yes ☐ No ☐	Yes ☐ No ☐				
	Yes ☐ No ☐	Yes ☐ No ☐				
	Yes ☐ No ☐	Yes ☐ No ☐				
	Yes ☐ No ☐	Yes ☐ No ☐				

9. Managing Open-Ended Tasks

Executive skills addressed: Emotional control (Chapter 13), flexibility (Chapter 19), metacognition (Chapter 21).

Ages: 7–14.

For many children, the most challenging homework assignment is one that involves an open-ended task. Open-ended tasks are those where (1) multiple correct answers are possible; (2) there are different ways to achieve the correct answer or desired result; (3) the task itself provides no clear feedback about its completion, leaving it to the child to decide when he or she is done; or (4) the task has no obvious starting point, leaving it to the child to decide what to do first.

Examples of open-ended tasks:

- Using spelling words in sentences
- Any writing assignment
- Showing several ways to solve a math problem (for example, "How many different ways can you group 24 items into even-numbered groups?")
- Selecting a strategy to solve a more complex math word problem
- Answering "Why?" questions
- Looking for answers to social studies questions in the text, unless the correct answer is one word or a concrete concept.

There are two ways to help children with open-ended tasks: (1) revise the tasks to make them more closed-ended or (2) teach them how to handle these kinds of tasks. Because problems handling open-ended tasks are most evident when children do open-ended homework assignments, it will be important to work with your child's teacher so that the teacher understands how difficult this is for your child (often the problems are more evident at home than at school) and why modifications need to be made.

Ways to make open-ended tasks more closed-ended:

- Talk your child through the task—either help him or her get started or talk about each step in the task and stay with your child while he or she performs each step.
- Don't ask your child to come up with ideas on his or her own—give him or her choices or narrow the number of choices. You may want to do this in consultation with your child's teacher so the teacher understands how—and why—the task is being modified. Over time, you can fade this modification—for instance, by gradually increasing the number of choices or by encouraging your child to add to the choices you're providing.

- Give your child "cheat sheets" or procedure lists (for example, the steps in a math process such as long division).
- Alter the task to remove the problem-solving demand. For instance, practice spelling words by writing each word 10 times rather than composing sentences or give your child sentences with the spelling words missing. Again, you'll want to make these modifications with the knowledge and approval of your child's teacher.
- Provide templates for writing assignments. The template itself then can walk the child through the task.
- Provide ample support in the prewriting phases—in particular, brainstorming ideas for writing assignments and organizing those ideas (see Writing a Paper).
- Ask your child's teacher to provide scoring rubrics that spell out exactly what is expected for any assignment.

The easiest way to help your child become more adept with open-ended tasks is to walk him or her through the task, using a think-aloud procedure. In other words, model the kinds of thoughts and strategies needed to attack the task. This generally involves providing close guidance and lots of support initially and then gradually fading the support, handing over the planning more and more to your child. For children with significant problems with flexibility, managing open-ended tasks successfully often takes years and thus may require assignment modifications and support by you and your child's teacher for a long time.

10. Long-Term Projects

Executive skills addressed: Task initiation (Chapter 15), sustained attention (Chapter 14), planning (Chapter 16), time management (Chapter 18), meta-cognition (Chapter 21).

Ages: 8–14; kids as young as 7 might be assigned such a project, but it will probably involve a simpler process, meaning this intervention should be simplified too.

1. With your child, look at the description of the assignment to make sure you both understand what is expected. If the assignment allows your child a choice of topic, topic selection is the first step. Many children have trouble thinking up topics, and if this is the case with your child, you should brainstorm topic ideas, providing lots of suggestions, starting with topics that are related to your child's areas of interests.

2. Using the Project Planning Sheet, write down the possible topics. After you have three to five, go back and ask your child what he or she likes and doesn't like about each choice.

3. Help your child make a final selection. In addition to thinking about what topic is of greatest interest, other things to think about in making a final selection are (a) choosing a topic that is neither too broad nor too narrow; (b) how difficult it will be to track down references and resources; and (c) whether there is an interesting "twist" to the topic that will either make it fun to work on or appealing for the teacher.

4. Using the Project Planning Sheet, decide what materials or resources will be needed, where the child will get them and when (you may want to fill in the last column after completing the next step). Possible resources include Internet websites, library books, things that may need to be ordered (for example, travel brochures), people that might be interviewed, or places to visit (for example, museums, historical sites, etc.). Also consider any construction or art materials that will be needed if the project involves building something.

5. Using the Project Planning Sheet, list all the steps that will need to be done to carry out the project and then develop a timeline so your child knows when each step will be done. It may be helpful at this point to transfer this information onto a monthly calendar that can be hung on the wall or a bulletin board near your child's desk to make it easier to keep track of what needs to be done when.

6. Cue your child to follow the timeline. Before he or she begins each step, you may want to have a discussion about what exactly is involved in completing the step—this may mean making a list of things to be done for each step. Planning for the next step could be done as each step is completed, so that your child has some idea what's coming next and to make it easier to get the next step started.

Fading the Supervision

Children who have problems with planning and with the metacognitive skills required to do open-ended tasks often require lots of support for a long time. Using the Project Planning Sheet as a guide, you can gradually hand over the responsibility of having your child complete the sheet more and more on his or her own. As you sense your child's ability to do more of the work independently, sit down with the planning sheet and have him or her indicate which pieces he or she thinks he or she can do alone and which pieces he or she will need help with. It is likely that you will continue to need to remind your child to complete each step in the timeline for a long time before the child can be independent in this part of the process.

Modifications/Adjustments

Use reinforcers as necessary for meeting timeline goals and for completing the project by the deadline; you can award bonus points for completion without reminders (or with a minimum, agreed-on number of reminders).

LONG-TERM PROJECT PLANNING SHEET

Step 1: Select Topic

What are possible topics?	What I like about this choice:	What I don't like:
1.		
2.		
3.		
4.		
5.		

Final topic choice:

Step 2: Identify Necessary Materials

What materials or resources do you need?	Where will you get them?	When will you get them?
1.		
2.		
3.		
4.		
5.		

Step 3: Identify Project Tasks and Due Dates

What do you need to do? (List each step in order)	When will you do it?	Check off when done
Step 1:		
Step 2:		
Step 3:		
Step 4:		
Step 5:		
Step 6:		
Step 7:		
Step 8:		
Step 9:		
Step 10:		

11. Writing a Paper

Executive skills addressed: Task initiation (Chapter 15), sustained attention (Chapter 14), planning (Chapter 16), organization (Chapter 17), time management (Chapter 18), metacognition (Chapter 21).

Ages: 8–14; children don't usually start writing papers till third grade, and they are typically shorter than five paragraphs for the youngest kids in this age range, so if your child is only 8, you may have to shorten the form accordingly.

Step 1: Brainstorm Topics

If your child has to come up with a topic to write about, you should make sure you understand the exact assignment requirements before beginning. This may necessitate a phone call to the teacher or a friend of your child to clarify directions. The rules of brainstorming are that any idea is accepted and written down in the first stage—the wilder and crazier, the better, because wild and crazy ideas often lead to good, usable ideas. No criticism by either parent or child is allowed at this point. If your child has trouble thinking of ideas on his or her own, throw out some ideas of your own to "grease the wheels." Once you and your child run out of topic ideas, read over your list and circle the most promising ones. Your child may know right away what he wants to write about. If not, talk about what he or she likes and dislikes about each idea to make it easier to zero in on a good choice.

Step 2: Brainstorm Content

Once a topic has been selected, the brainstorming process begins again. Ask your child, "Tell me everything you know or would like to know about this topic." Again, write down any idea or question, the crazier the better at this point.

Step 3: Organize the Content

Now look at all the ideas or questions you've written down. Together with your child, decide whether the material can be grouped together in any way. If the assignment is to do a report on aardvarks, for instance, you might find the information clusters into categories such as what they look like, where they live, what they eat, who their enemies are, how they protect themselves. Create topic headings and then write the details under each topic heading. Some parents find that it's helpful to use Post-its for this process. During the brainstorming phase, each individual idea or question is written on a separate Post-It. The Post-Its can then be organized on a table under topic headings to form an outline of the paper. The paper can then be written (or dictated) from this outline.

Step 4: Write the Opening Paragraph

This is often the hardest part of the paper to write. The opening paragraph, at its most basic level, describes very succinctly what the paper will be about. For instance, an opening paragraph on a report about aardvarks might read:

> This paper is about a strange animal called an aardvark. By the time you finish reading it, you will know what they look like, where they live, what they eat, who their enemies are, and how they protect themselves.

The one other thing that the opening paragraph should try to do is "grab the reader"—give the reader an interesting piece of information to tease his or her curiosity. At the end of the paragraph above, for instance, two more sentences might be added:

> The reader will also learn the meaning of the word aardvark and what language it comes from. And if that hasn't grabbed your interest, I will also tell you why the aardvark has a sticky tongue—although you may not want to know this!

Children with writing problems will have trouble writing the opening paragraph by themselves and may need your help. You may be able to help by asking general questions, such as "What do you want people to know after they read your paper?" or "Why do you think people might be interested in reading this?" If they need more help than that, you may want to give them a model to work from. You could write an opening paragraph on a topic similar to the one your child is working on, or you could use the paragraph here as an example. If your child needs more guided help writing this paragraph, provide it. Then see if he or she can continue without the need for as much support. Remember, the first paragraph is often the hardest part of the paper to write.

Step 5: Write the Rest of the Paper

To give your child just a little more guidance, suggest that the rest of the paper be divided into sections with a heading for each section (sort of the way this manual is written). Help him or her make a list of the headings and then see if he or she can continue with the writing task alone. Each paragraph should begin with a main or topic sentence that makes one main point. Following the topic sentence should be three to five sentences that expand or explain the main point. It's helpful to use connecting words to link sentences or paragraphs. Examples of simple linking words are *and, because, also, instead, but, so.* Examples of more complex linking words are *although, moreover, on the other hand, therefore, as a result, finally, in conclusion.*

In the early stages of learning to write, children with writing problems need a great deal of help. You may feel like you're writing half the paper in the early stages. It should get better with time, especially if you end each writing session by giving your child some positive feedback about something done well. Note in particular any improvement since the last writing assignment. You might say, "I really like the way you were able to come up with the headings on your own this time, with no help from me."

If you don't see progress over time—or if you feel you lack the time or skills to teach your child to do this kind of writing, talk with your child's teacher to see if additional support can be provided in school. Even if you're willing to help out in this way, you may want to ask for more help in school if you believe your child's writing skills are significantly delayed compared to other children of the same age.

WRITING TEMPLATE FOR A FIVE-PARAGRAPH ESSAY

Introductory paragraph

Sentence 1 summarizes what your essay is about:

Sentence 2 focuses in on the main point you want to make:

Sentence 3 adds more detail or explains why the topic is important:

Body paragraphs

Paragraph 1, topic sentence:

   Supporting detail 1:

   Supporting detail 2:

   Supporting detail 3:

Paragraph 2, topic sentence:

   Supporting detail 1:

   Supporting detail 2:

   Supporting detail 3:

Paragraph 3, topic sentence:

   Supporting detail 1:

   Supporting detail 2:

   Supporting detail 3:

Concluding paragraph

Restate the most important point from the paper you want to make (what the reader should go away understanding):

From *Smart but Scattered* by Peg Dawson and Richard Guare. Copyright 2009 by The Guilford Press.

12. Studying for Tests

Executive skills addressed: Task initiation (Chapter 15), sustained attention (Chapter 14), planning (Chapter 16), time management (Chapter 18), metacognition (Chapter 21).

Ages: 10–14; children usually don't have tests till fourth grade, and even then the teacher is likely to tell them what to study, so this routine probably won't be of much use to you until your child is in at least fifth grade.

1. Keep a monthly calendar with your child on which any upcoming tests are written.
2. From 5 days to a week before the test, make a study plan with your child.
3. Using the Menu of Study Strategies, have your child decide which strategies he or she wants to use to study for the test.
4. Have your child make a plan for studying that starts 4 days before the test. Psychological research over many years shows that when new material is learned, *distributed practice is more effective than massed practice*. In other words, if you plan to spend 2 hours studying for a test, it is better to break the time down into smaller segments (such as 30 minutes a night for 4 nights) than to spend the full 2 hours studying the night before the test. Research also shows that learning is consolidated through sleep, so getting a good night's sleep the night before an exam is more beneficial than "cramming" the night before.
5. For children who have problems with sustained attention, using several strategies each for a short amount of time may be easier than using one strategy for the full study period. You can set a kitchen timer for the length of time for each strategy, and when the bell rings, your child can move on to the next strategy (unless the child likes the one being used and wants to continue it).

Fading the Supervision

Depending on your child's level of independence, he or she may need help making the study plan, may need prompting to follow the plan, and may need supervision while he or she is following the plan. You can gradually fade this support, first by having your child check in with you after he's finished each strategy, but keeping all the other supports in place. Cueing to make the study plan and prompting to start studying will likely be the last supports you can fade.

Modifications/Adjustments

1. After your child takes the test or after the graded test is returned, ask your child to evaluate how the study plan went. Which strategies seemed to work the best? Which ones were less helpful? Are there other strategies he or she might try the

next time? How about the time devoted to studying? Was it enough? Make some notes on the study plan to help your child when it's time to plan for the next test.

2. If your child felt he or she studied adequately, but still did poorly, check with his or her teacher for feedback about what might have been done differently. Did your child study the wrong material—or study it in the wrong way? Consider asking your child's teacher to prepare a study guide, if that hasn't been done already.

3. If your child consistently does poorly on tests despite studying long and hard, consider asking his or her teacher for testing modifications (for example, extended time, the chance to retake tests, the chance to do extra credit work to make up for poor test grades, alternatives to tests, or allowing your child to prepare a cheat sheet or take open-book exams). This may require that your child be evaluated to determine whether he or she qualifies for special education services or a 504 Plan (discussed in Chapter 23).

4. Add an incentive system—rewards for good grades on tests.

MENU OF STUDY STRATEGIES

Check off the ones you will use.

___ 1. Reread text	___ 2. Reread/organize notes	___ 3. Read/recite main points
___ 4. Outline text	___ 5. Highlight text	___ 6. Highlight notes
___ 7. Use study guide	___ 8. Make concept maps	___ 9. Make lists/ organize
___ 10. Take practice test	___ 11. Quiz myself	___ 12. Have someone else quiz me
___ 13. Study flash cards	___ 14. Memorize/ rehearse	___ 15. Create a "cheat sheet"
___ 16. Study with friend	___ 17. Study with study group	___ 18. Study session with teacher
___ 19. Study with a parent	___ 20. Ask for help	___ 21. Other: _____

STUDY PLAN

Date	Day	Which strategies will I use? (write #)	How much time for each strategy?
	4 days before test	1. _____ 2. _____ 3. _____	1. _____ 2. _____ 3. _____
	3 days before test	1. _____ 2. _____ 3. _____	1. _____ 2. _____ 3. _____
	2 days before test	1. _____ 2. _____ 3. _____	1. _____ 2. _____ 3. _____
	1 day before test	1. _____ 2. _____ 3. _____	1. _____ 2. _____ 3. _____

Posttest Evaluation

How did your studying work out? Answer the following questions:

1. What strategies worked best?

2. What strategies were not so helpful?

3. Did you spend enough time studying? ❑ Yes ❑ No

4. If no, what more should you have done?

5. What will you do differently the next time?

13. Learning to Manage Tasks That Take Lots of Effort

Executive skills addressed: Task initiation (Chapter 15), sustained attention (Chapter 14).

Ages: Any age.

There are two primary ways to make tasks that your child sees as taking a lot of effort less aversive to the child: Cut down the amount of effort required, by making it briefer or easier, or offer a large enough incentive that the child is willing to expend the effort required to get the reward. Examples of ways to do this are:

1. Break the task down into very small parts, so that each part requires no more than 5 minutes. Allow your child to earn a small reward at the end of each part.
2. Allow your child to decide how to break down the task. For example, make a list of homework activities or chores and let your child decide how much of each task will be done before he or she earns a break.
3. Give your child something powerful to look forward to doing when the task is done. For instance, your child might earn 45 minutes of video game time for completing his nightly homework (and/or chores), without complaining, within a specified time frame, and with an agreed-on quality (such as making no more than one mistake on the math homework).
4. Reward your child for being willing to tackle tasks that demand effort. You could, for example, draw up a chore list and have your child rate each chore for effort required. Then you could assign a larger reward (such as more video game time) for choosing to do the harder chores. It may be helpful to create a scale for effort—1 for the easiest tasks up to 10 for the hardest tasks your child could ever imagine doing. Once your child masters the use of the scale, you could work on thinking about how to turn a high-effort task (say, one rated 8–10) into a lower effort task (one rated 3–4).

Modifications/Adjustments

If approaches such as these don't help your child complete tough tasks without complaining, whining, crying, or otherwise resisting, you may want to take a slower and more labor-intensive approach to training your child to tolerate high-effort tasks. This approach, mentioned earlier under Bedroom Cleaning, is called *backward chaining*. Essentially your child starts at the end of a high-effort task, at first completing only the very last step to earn a reward. For bedroom cleaning, this last step might be having the child put the dirty clothes in the laundry after you've tidied the rest of the child's room or having him put what he needs for the schoolday into his backpack after you've assisted him through the earlier steps of his morning routine.

You keep repeating this process until your child can do that one step easily and effortlessly. Then you back up one step and require the child to do only the last *two* steps in the task before earning the reward. Over time, your child is backed through the task until you get to the point where you expect him to complete the entire task independently. Many parents resist this approach, especially if they know that the child will eventually clean his room if they nag and harass him long enough. But who wants to have to nag for the rest of their parental life? Backward chaining actually trains the child to tolerate tedious or high-effort work and eventually eliminates the need for nagging.

14. Organizing Notebooks/Homework

Executive skills addressed: Organization (Chapter 17), task initiation (Chapter 15).

Ages: 6–14.

1. With your child, decide on what needs to be included in the organizational system: A place to keep unfinished homework? A separate place to keep completed homework? A place to keep papers that need to be filed? Notebooks or binders to keep notes, completed assignments, handouts, worksheets, etc.? A sample list is in the checklist that follows.
2. Once you've listed all these elements, decide how best to handle them, one at a time. For example, you and your child might decide on a colored folder system, with a different color for completed assignments, unfinished work, and other papers. Or you might decide to have a separate small three-ring binder for each subject or one large binder to handle all subjects. You may want to visit an office supply store to gather ideas.
3. Gather the materials you need—from the house if you have them on hand or from the office supply store if you don't. Materials should include a three-hole punch, lined and unlined paper, subject dividers, and small Post-it packages your child might want to use to flag important papers.
4. Set up the notebooks and folders, labeling everything clearly.
5. At the beginning of each homework session, have your child take out the folders for completed assignments, unfinished work, and material to be filed. Have your child make a decision about each piece of material and where it should go. Complete this process before beginning homework.
6. When homework is completed, have your child place homework in the appropriate folder and file anything else that needs to be saved.

Fading the Supervision

1. Cue your child to begin homework by following the "organizing" process. Supervise each step of the process to make sure all steps are followed and checked off on a checklist.
2. Cue your child to begin homework with the organizing process and remind him or her to check off each step when done. Check back periodically and check in at the end of homework to make sure the checklist is done and that materials have been stored appropriately.
3. Cue at the beginning, check in at the end, and do occasional spot checks of notebooks, folders, and other files.

Modifications/Adjustments

1. As much as possible, involve your child in the design of the organizing system. We've discovered that what works well for one person is a disaster for another because it's not a good fit.
2. Redesign the elements that aren't working right. Again, involve your child in the troubleshooting. "How could this work better for you?" is the way to approach this.
3. For people who are not naturally organized, it can take a long time for this process to become a habit. Keep in mind that supervision over the long haul may be necessary.

SETTING UP A NOTEBOOK/HOMEWORK MANAGEMENT SYSTEM

System element	What will you use?	Got it (✓)
Place for unfinished homework		
Place for completed assignments		
Place to keep materials for later filing		
Notebooks or binder(s) for each subject		
Other things you might need: 1. 2. 3. 4.		

From *Smart but Scattered* by Peg Dawson and Richard Guare. Copyright 2009 by The Guilford Press.

MAINTAINING A NOTEBOOK/HOMEWORK MANAGEMENT SYSTEM

Task	Monday	Tuesday	Wednesday	Thursday	Weekend
Clean out "to be filed" folder					
Go through notebooks and books for other loose papers and file them					
Do homework					
Place all assignments (both finished and unfinished) in appropriate places					

From *Smart but Scattered* by Peg Dawson and Richard Guare. Copyright 2009 by The Guilford Press.

15. Learning to Control His or Her Temper

Executive skills addressed: Emotional control (Chapter 13), response inhibition (Chapter 11), flexibility (Chapter 19).

Ages: Any age.

1. Together with your child, make a list of the things that happen that cause your child to lose his or her temper (these are called *triggers*). You may want to make a long list of all the different things that make your child angry and then see if they can be grouped into larger categories (when told "no," when he or she loses a game, when something promised doesn't happen, etc.).
2. Talk with your child about what "losing your temper looks or sounds like" (for example, yells, swears, throws things, kicks things or people, etc.). Decide which ones of these should go on a "can't do" list. Keep this list short and work on only one or two behaviors at a time.
3. Now make a list of things your child can do instead (called *replacement behaviors*). These should be three or four different things your child can do instead of the "can't do" behaviors you've selected.
4. Put these on a "Hard Times Board" (see the example that follows).
5. Practice. Say to your child, "Let's pretend you're upset because Billy said he would come over to play and then he had to do something else instead. Which strategy do you want to use?" (See the more detailed practice guidelines that follow.)
6. After practicing for a couple of weeks, start using the process "for real," but initially use it for only minor irritants.
7. After using it successfully with minor irritants, move on to the more challenging triggers.
8. Connect the process to a reward. For best results, use two levels of rewards: a "big reward" for never getting to the point where the Hard Times Board needs to be used, and a "small reward" for successfully using a strategy on the Hard Times Board to deal with the trigger situation.

Practicing the Procedure

1. Use real-life examples. These should include a variety representing the different categories of triggers.
2. Make the practice sessions "quick and dirty." For example, if a coping strategy is to read a book, have your child open a book and start reading, but don't spend more than 20–30 seconds on this.
3. Have your child practice each of the strategies listed on the Hard Times Board.
4. Have brief practice sessions daily or several times a week for a couple of weeks before putting it into effect.

Modifications/Adjustments

1. At first you may need to model the use of the strategy. This means talking aloud to show what your child might be saying or thinking as he or she implements the strategy.
2. There may be times when, despite having a procedure in place, your child still loses control and can't calm down or use any of the strategies on the Hard Times Board. In this case, remove the child from the situation (physically if necessary). Tell the child in advance that you will do this, so that your child knows what to expect. Say, "If you hit or kick or scream, we're always going to leave."
3. If your child is fairly consistently unable to use the strategies effectively, it may be time to consider seeking professional help; see Chapter 22.

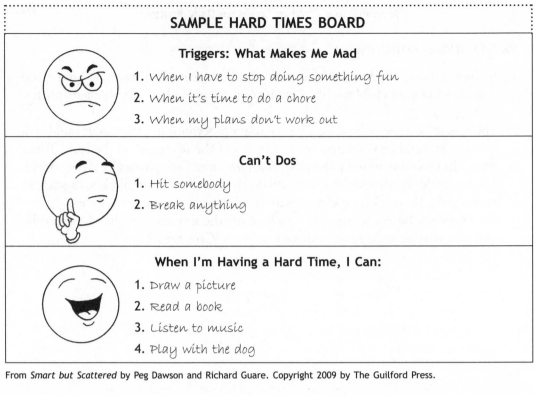

SAMPLE HARD TIMES BOARD

Triggers: What Makes Me Mad

1. When I have to stop doing something fun
2. When it's time to do a chore
3. When my plans don't work out

Can't Dos

1. Hit somebody
2. Break anything

When I'm Having a Hard Time, I Can:

1. Draw a picture
2. Read a book
3. Listen to music
4. Play with the dog

From *Smart but Scattered* by Peg Dawson and Richard Guare. Copyright 2009 by The Guilford Press.

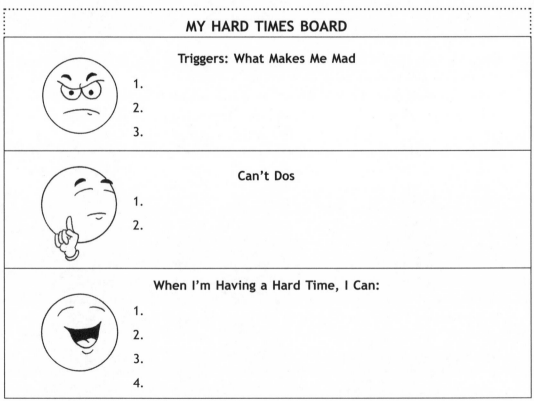

MY HARD TIMES BOARD

Triggers: What Makes Me Mad

1.
2.
3.

Can't Dos

1.
2.

When I'm Having a Hard Time, I Can:

1.
2.
3.
4.

From *Smart but Scattered* by Peg Dawson and Richard Guare. Copyright 2009 by The Guilford Press.

16. Learning to Control Impulsive Behavior

Executive skills addressed: Response inhibition (Chapter 11), emotional control (Chapter 13).

Ages: Any age.

1. Together with your child, identify the triggers for the impulsive behavior (watching TV with siblings, open-ended play with friends, or whatever).
2. Agree on a rule for the trigger situation. The rule should focus on what your child can do to control impulses. Build in choice if you can—in other words, you and your child should come up with a couple of different things he or she can do in place of the unwanted impulsive response.
3. Talk about what you might do to signal to your child that you think he or she is on the verge of "losing control" so that he or she can back off or use one of the coping strategies agreed on. This works best when the signal is a relatively discrete visual signal (for example, a hand motion) that can alert your child to the problem situation.
4. Practice the procedure. Make this a "Let's pretend" role-play. "Let's pretend you're outside playing with your friends and one of them says something that makes you mad. I'll be your friend and you be you." If this is hard for your child, you may want to play your child in this role-play to model how he or she will handle the situation.
5. As with the other skills involving behavior regulation, practice the procedure daily or several times a week for a couple of weeks.
6. When you and your child are ready to put the procedure in effect in "real life," remind him or her about it just before the trigger situation is likely to occur (for example, "Remember the plan," "Remember what we talked about").
7. Review how the process worked afterward. You may want to create a scale that you and your child can use to assess how well it went (5—Went without a hitch! to 1—*That* didn't go real well!).

Modifications/Adjustments

1. If you think it will make the process work more effectively or more quickly, tie the successful use of a replacement behavior to a reinforcer. This may best be done using a "response cost" approach. For example, give your child 70 points to begin the day. Each time your child acts impulsively, subtract 10 points. You can also give bonus points if your child gets through a specified period of time without losing any points.
2. If impulsivity is a significant problem for your child, begin by choosing one time of day or one impulsive behavior to target to make success more likely.
3. Be sure to praise your child for showing self-control. Even if you're using tangible rewards, social praise should always accompany any other kind of reinforcer.

The things I do without thinking include:

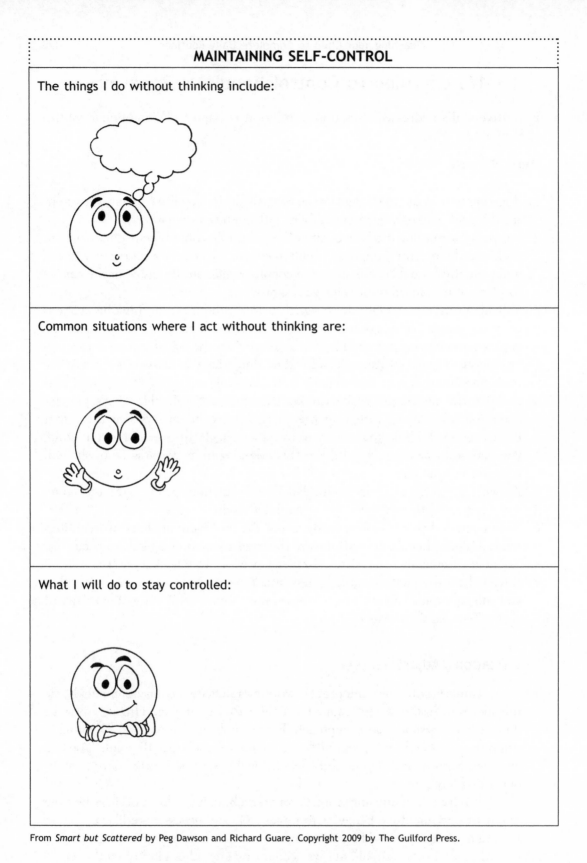

Common situations where I act without thinking are:

What I will do to stay controlled:

17. Learning to Manage Anxiety

Executive skills addressed: Emotional control (Chapter 13), flexibility (Chapter 19).

Ages: All ages.

1. Together with your child, make a list of the things that happen that cause your child to feel anxious. See if there's a pattern and whether different situations can be grouped into one larger category (for example, a child who gets nervous on the soccer field, when giving an oral report in school, and playing in a piano recital may have *performance* anxiety—that is, he or she gets nervous when he or she has to perform in front of others).
2. Talk with your child about what anxiety feels like so he or she can recognize it in the early stages. This is often a physical feeling—"butterflies" in the stomach, sweaty hands, faster heartbeat.
3. Now make a list of things your child can do instead of thinking about the worry (called *replacement behaviors*). These should be three or four different things your child can do that either are calming or divert attention from the worries.
4. Put these on a "Worry Board" (an example follows).
5. Practice. Say to your child, "Let's pretend you're getting nervous because you have a baseball tryout and you're worried you won't make the team. Which strategy do you want to use?" (See the more detailed practice guidelines that follow.)
6. After practicing for a couple of weeks, start using the process "for real" but initially use it for only minor worries.
7. After using it successfully with minor worries, move on to bigger anxieties.
8. Connect the process to a reward. For best results, use two levels of rewards: a "big reward" for never getting to the point where the Worry Board needs to be used and a "small reward" for successfully using a strategy on the Worry Board to deal with the trigger situation.

Practicing the Procedure

1. Use real-life examples. These should include a variety representing the different categories of triggers.
2. Make the practice sessions "quick and dirty." For example, if a coping strategy is to practice "thought stopping," have the child practice the following self-talk strategy: Tell her to say, loudly and forcefully (but to herself), "STOP!" This momentarily interrupts any thought. As soon the child has done this, have her think of a pleasant image or scene. Practice this a few times daily. When the problem or anxiety-provoking thought occurs, use this strategy and continue repeating it until the thought stops.

3. Have your child practice each of the strategies listed on the Worry Board.
4. Have brief practice sessions daily or several times a week for a couple of weeks before putting it into effect.

Modifications/Adjustments

1. Possible coping strategies for managing anxiety might include deep or slow breathing, counting to 20, using other relaxation strategies, thought stopping or talking back to your worries, drawing a picture of the worry, folding it up, and putting it in a box with a lid, listening to music (and maybe dancing to it), challenging the logic of the worry. For further explanation for these, type "relaxation for kids" into a search engine and check out the websites that come up. Another helpful resource is a book written for children and parents to read together: *What to Do When You Worry Too Much* by Dawn Huebner, PhD.
2. Helping children manage anxiety generally involves a procedure sometimes called *desensitization* in which the degree of anxiety to which the child is exposed is low enough so that with some support he or she can get through it successfully. For example, if a child is afraid of dogs, you might begin by asking him to look at a picture of a dog and model what he might say to himself ("I'm looking at this picture, and it's a little scary when I think of there being a real dog, but I'm managing okay, I'm not getting too scared. I can look at the picture okay."). The next step might be to have the child be inside a house with a dog outside and talk about what that's like. Very gradually, bring the dog closer to the child. A similar approach can be used with other fears and phobias. The exposure has to be very gradual; you don't move to the next step until the child feels comfortable with the current step. The critical elements in guided mastery are physical distance and time—in the beginning, the child is far removed from the anxiety-provoking object and the exposure is for a very short time. The distance is then reduced and the time increased gradually. It's also helpful to have a script (something the child is to say in the situation) and a tactic he can use (such as thought stopping or something he can do to divert his attention).
3. The kinds of worries or anxieties that this approach will work with are (1) separation anxiety (being unhappy or worried when separated from a loved one, usually a parent); (2) handling novel or unfamiliar situations; and (3) obsessive or catastrophic thinking (worrying about something bad happening). This approach should work with all three, although the coping strategies for each may vary.

SAMPLE WORRY BOARD

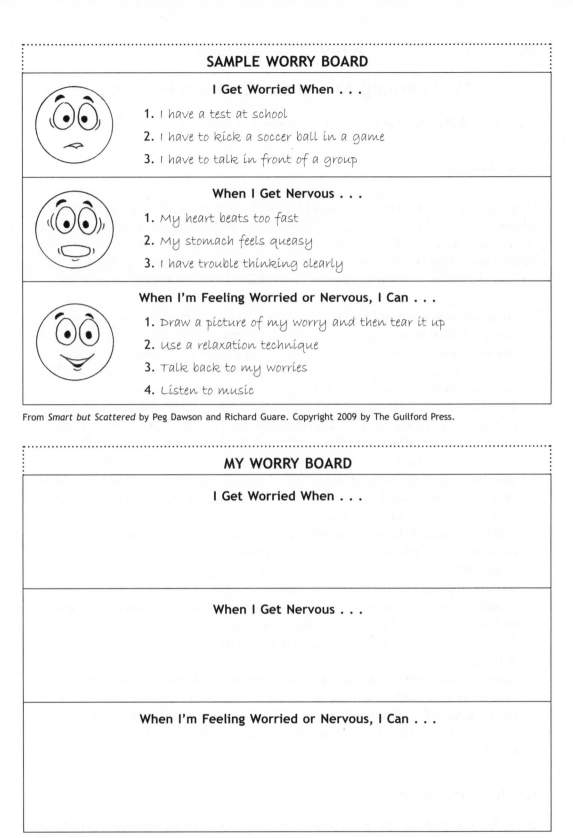

I Get Worried When . . .

1. I have a test at school
2. I have to kick a soccer ball in a game
3. I have to talk in front of a group

When I Get Nervous . . .

1. My heart beats too fast
2. My stomach feels queasy
3. I have trouble thinking clearly

When I'm Feeling Worried or Nervous, I Can . . .

1. Draw a picture of my worry and then tear it up
2. Use a relaxation technique
3. Talk back to my worries
4. Listen to music

MY WORRY BOARD

I Get Worried When . . .

When I Get Nervous . . .

When I'm Feeling Worried or Nervous, I Can . . .

18. Learning to Handle Changes in Plans

Executive skills addressed: Emotional control (Chapter 13), flexibility (Chapter 19).

Ages: Any age.

Helping your child accept changes in plans without anger or distress involves some advance work and lots of practice. Whenever possible, you need to present your agenda for your child ahead of time, before the child has formulated his or her own plan for that time period. Meanwhile, you start introducing the child to small changes on a regular basis, gradually increasing the child's tolerance for surprises over time.

1. Sit down with your child and establish a schedule of activities and tasks. This might mean creating some organization and routine for the day, or it might mean simply making a list of events that are already part of a routine. Include any activity that is a "have to" as far as you're concerned (mealtimes, bedtime, etc.) and any regular activity (such as lessons and sports).
2. Try not to attach precise times to the activities unless necessary (as with sports events and lessons), using time ranges instead. For example, dinner might be around 5:00 P.M., which could be between 4:30 and 5:30.
3. Talk with your child about the fact that changes or "surprises" can always come up despite plans and schedules established in advance. Give examples: instead of fish, we have pizza for dinner; you get to play outside for an extra 20 minutes; we have to go to the dentist today.
4. Create a visual for the schedule, such as activities written on a card or a series of pictures, and post it in at least two places, such as the kitchen and your child's room. Make a "Surprise!" card for the schedule and explain that when a change is coming, you will show him the card, say what the change is, and put it on the schedule. (Even when a change comes up that's a surprise to everyone, you can pull out the card and follow the same process.)
5. Review the schedule with your child either the night before and/or the morning of the day.
6. Start to introduce changes and show the Surprise card. Initially, these should be pleasant, such as extra playtime, going out for ice cream, playing a game with a parent. Gradually introduce more "neutral" changes (apple juice for orange juice, one cereal for another, etc.) Eventually, include less pleasant changes (can't do a planned activity because of weather).

Modifications/Adjustments

If the Surprise card and the gradual introduction of changes are not sufficient, there are a few other approaches to consider. When possible, introduce the change well before the event. This gives your child time to adjust gradually rather than quickly. Depending on his or her reaction to less pleasant change (crying, resisting, complaining), talk about other behaviors the child could use that would allow for protest in an acceptable way (such as filling out a Complaint Form). You also can provide a reward for successfully managing the change. Keep in mind that reactivity to change decreases with the amount of exposure that the child has and the success he has in negotiating it. As long as the exposure is gradual and does not initially involve situations that are frustrating or threatening, your child can become more flexible.

MANAGING CHANGES IN PLANS OR SCHEDULES

Daily Schedule

Date: _____

Time	Activity

Surprise:

Complaint Form

Date: _____

Nature of complaint:

Why you think the situation was unfair:

What you wish had happened:

19. Learning Not to Cry over Little Things

Executive skills addressed: Emotional control (Chapter 13), flexibility (Chapter 19).

Ages: Any age.

When children cry over little things, they're generally trying to communicate that they want sympathy, and they're using this method of getting it because they've found it effective in the past. So the goal of this intervention is not to teach kids to be tough little soldiers or anything of the sort, but to help them find ways other than crying to get what they want. The goal is to get them to use words instead of tears in those situations where crying does not appear to be an appropriate response.

1. Let your child know that crying too much makes people disinclined to spend time with him or her and that you want to help the child find other ways of handling feelings when upset so that this doesn't happen.
2. Explain that your child needs to use words instead of tears when upset. This can be done by having your child label his or her feelings ("I'm upset," "I'm sad," "I'm angry," etc.).
3. Let your child know that it may be helpful for him or her to explain what caused these feelings (for example, "I'm upset because I was hoping to go to Joey's house, but when I called, no one was home," or "I'm mad because I lost the game").
4. When your child is able to use words, respond by validating his or her feelings (for example, "I can see you're upset. Not being able to play with a friend must be a big disappointment to you"). Statements like this will communicate to the child that you understand and sympathize.
5. Let your child know in advance what will happen when an upsetting situation arrives. This should include giving him or her a script for handling the situation. You might say, "When you feel like crying, you can use words like 'I'm angry,' 'I'm sad,' 'I need help,' or 'I need a break.' When you use words, I'll listen and try to understand your feelings. If you start to cry, though, you're on your own. I'll either leave the room or ask you to go to your bedroom to finish crying." At first you may periodically need to remind your child of the procedure to prepare him or her to follow the script when an upsetting situation occurs.
6. As soon as your child starts to cry, make sure he or she gets no attention from anyone for crying. This means no attention from *anyone* (siblings, parents, grandparents, etc.), so you should make sure everybody likely to be involved understands the procedure. Without the attention for crying, it will gradually diminish (although it may get worse initially before it gets better).
7. The goal here is not to extinguish *all crying* (because there are legitimate reasons for children to cry). A rule of thumb for judging when it may be appropriate to cry is to think about the average child of your child's age. Would crying be a nat-

ural response in the situation at hand? Crying is appropriate, for instance, when dealing with physical pain or when a serious misfortune befalls your child or someone your child is close to.

Modifications/Adjustments

If crying is firmly entrenched, you may want to build in a reinforcer to help your child learn to use words instead of tears. Depending on the age of your child, you could give him or her stickers or points for using words instead of tears or for going a certain amount of time without crying. To determine how long that time should be, it would be helpful to take a baseline so you know how frequently your child cries now. A log to help you track how often the crying occurs, how long it lasts, and what the precipitating event is is included to help you do this. Following it is a "contract" you can make with your child to handle crying. Depending on the age of the child, the contract can be completed with words, pictures, or both.

UPSET LOG

Date	Time	Duration of upset	Precipitating event

Here's what I can do instead of crying:

Here's what will happen if I can keep from crying when I'm upset:

Here's what will happen when I cry over little things:

20. Learning to Solve Problems

Executive skills addressed: metacognition (Chapter 21), flexibility (Chapter 19).

Ages: 7–14; even though metacognition in its most advanced form is one of the latest skills to develop, you can do problem solving with younger kids too (see, for example, the widely respected program called *I Can Problem Solve*, by Myrna B. Shure, PhD, for preschoolers).

1. Talk with your child about what the problem is. This generally involves three steps: (a) empathizing with the child or letting the child know you understand how he or she feels ("I can see that makes you really mad" or "That must be really upsetting for you"); (b) getting a *general* sense of what the problem is ("Let me get this straight—you're upset because the friend you were hoping to play with can't come over"); and (c) defining the problem more narrowly so that you can begin to brainstorm solutions ("You have a whole afternoon free, and you can't figure out what to do").
2. Brainstorm solutions. Together with your child, think of as many different things as you can that might solve the problem. You may want to set a time limit (like 2 minutes) because this sometimes speeds up the process or makes it feel less like an open-ended task. Write down all the possible solutions. Don't criticize the solutions at this point because this tends to squelch the creative thinking process.
3. Ask your child to look at all the solutions and pick the one he or she likes best. You may want to start by having him or her circle the top three to five choices and then narrow them down by talking about the pluses and minuses associated with each choice.
4. Ask your child if he or she needs help carrying out the choice.
5. Talk about what will happen if the first solution doesn't work. This may involve choosing a different solution or analyzing where the first solution went wrong and fixing it.
6. Praise him or her for coming up with a good solution (and then praise again after the solution is implemented).

Modifications/Adjustments

This is a standard problem-solving approach that can be used for all kinds of problems, including interpersonal problems as well as obstacles that prevent a child from getting what he or she wants or needs. Sometimes the best solution will involve figuring out ways to overcome the obstacles, while at other times it may involve helping your child come to terms with the fact that he or she cannot have what he or she wants.

Sometimes the problem-solving process may lead to a "negotiation," where you and your child agree on what will be done to reach a solution that's satisfactory. In this case, you should explain to your child that whatever solution you come up with, you both have to be able to live with it. You may want to talk about how labor contracts are negotiated so that both workers and bosses get something they want out of the bargain.

After you've used the process (and the worksheet) with your child for a number of different kinds of problems, your child may be able to use the worksheet independently. Because your goal should be to foster independent problem solving, you may want to ask your child to fill out the Solving Problems Worksheet alone before coming to you for your help (if needed). Eventually, your child will internalize the whole process and be able to solve problems "on the fly."

SOLVING PROBLEMS WORKSHEET

What is my problem?

What are some possible things I could do to solve my problem?

What will I try first?

If this doesn't work, what can I do?

How did it go? Did my solution work?

What might I do differently the next time?

11

Building Response Inhibition

Response inhibition is the capacity to think before you act—to resist the urge to say or do something before you've had a chance to evaluate the situation. In adults, the *absence* of this skill is more apparent to the casual observer than the presence of the skill because most of us maintain a level of self-control that enables us to function well at home and at work. Most of us have learned on the long road to adulthood, often through painful experience, how to think before acting. When we spot someone who does stand out due to a lack of response inhibition, we have a multitude of metaphors and other expressions to describe the behavior that results: we say the person "shoots from the hip" or "flies off the handle," or we just comment "open mouth, insert foot."

Some of us exercise this executive skill quite well until we find ourselves in an emotionally charged situation. In this day of instant communication, angry emails that the sender instantly regrets—or regrets after receiving an equally angry response—are a common product of poor response inhibition. Our ability to think before acting also suffers when we're physically impaired by too much alcohol, too little sleep, or too much stress. If you tend to jump to conclusions, or you act before you have all the necessary facts, or you blurt out whatever pops into your mind without thinking, you may lack response inhibition yourself. To help your child overcome a lack of response inhibition when you share the weakness, see the suggestions in Chapter 3.

How Response Inhibition Develops

As we said early in this book, response inhibition emerges first in infancy. In its most rudimentary form, response inhibition allows an infant to "choose" to respond or not respond to whatever is before the baby. Prior to its emergence, babies are pretty much at the mercy of their environment. If something enters their visual field, they're obligated to fixate on it, at least long enough to make sense out of it. With response inhibition comes the capacity to ignore or not be deterred by interruptions if there's something else they are working toward. Once language develops, the capacity to inhibit responding becomes more developed because they can internalize rules given to them by others (for example, "Don't touch the hot stove").

Just as goal-directed persistence, in its most advanced and complex form, may be the culminating executive skill that defines a mature adult, response inhibition is the fundamental executive skill that enables all other executive skills to develop. A child at the mercy of his impulses can't initiate, sustain attention, plan, organize, or problem solve effectively. One who develops a strong ability to inhibit his impulses has a significant advantage in school, making friends, and ultimately setting and achieving goals.

A famous study conducted many years ago showed that kids vary in their ability to inhibit responses when very young and that those variations predict different levels of success later in development. Three-year-olds were left alone in a room with one marshmallow and given the choice of eating it or waiting until the scientist returned and getting two marshmallows. Through a one-way mirror, the researchers watched some of the children control their impulse to eat the single marshmallow by talking to themselves, avoiding looking at the marshmallow, or finding other ways to divert their attention from the candy. When the researchers followed up many years later, they found that those children who had good response inhibition as 3-year-olds were earning better grades on their report cards, were less likely to be in trouble with the law, and were more successful in other ways.

While children become more adept at using most executive skills over time and with age, the development of response inhibition may not follow so steady a trajectory. Response inhibition, it seems, may be more susceptible to disruption in adolescence. Neuroscientists studying how the brain changes during the teen years have found that there is something of a "disconnect" between the lower centers of the brain, where emotions and impulses are processed, and the prefrontal cortex, where rational decisions are made. Only slowly, over the course of adolescence, and even into adulthood, do these connections become stronger and faster (through pruning and myelination, as described in Chapter 1), enabling young people to temper their emotions with reason. Until those connections are firmly in place, youngsters are likely to make decisions rashly and based on "gut feelings" without the anchoring influence of sound judgment that the frontal lobes provide.

Meanwhile, teenagers are undergoing other developmental changes that challenge impulse control. Gaining autonomy is a critical developmental task that's facilitated when teens become more strongly influenced by their peers and at the same time begin to challenge parental authority. Unfortunately, while this shift is helping teens become independent, it's also potentially making the teens more impulsive. And to make matters even more complicated, society as a whole starts to loosen the controls, allowing teenagers a lot more freedom in how they spend their time and who they spend it with. Inevitably, this loosening of control, as essential as it is, can lead to bad decisions. If we're lucky, bad decisions will result in good lessons learned and no permanent damage to our children or anybody else. But we can increase our luck in this area if we actively help our children learn to control their impulses.

How does your child's ability to control her impulses stack up against what's developmentally appropriate? The rating scale in the questionnaire below can help you answer this question, confirming or denying your preliminary assessment from Chapter 2 by giving you the chance to look a little more closely at how often your child is able to use this skill.

HOW WELL CAN YOUR CHILD INHIBIT IMPULSES?

Use the following scale to rate how well your child performs each of the tasks listed. At each level, children can be expected to perform all the tasks listed fairly well to very well.

Scale

0—Never or rarely

1—Does but not well (about 25% of the time)

2—Does fairly well (about 75% of the time)

3—Does very well (always or almost always)

Preschool/kindergarten

_____ Acts appropriately in situations where danger is obvious (e.g., not running into the road to retrieve a ball, looking both ways before crossing street)

_____ Can share toys without grabbing

_____ Can wait for a short period of time when instructed by an adult

Lower elementary (grades 1-3)

_____ Can follow simple classroom rules (e.g., raising hand before speaking)

_____ Can be in close proximity to another child without need for physical contact

_____ Can wait until a parent gets off the phone before telling the parent something (may need reminders)

Upper elementary (grades 4-5)

_____ Handles conflict with peers without getting into physical fights (may lose temper)

(cont.)

_____ Follows home or school rules without an adult's immediate presence

_____ Can calm down or de-escalate from emotionally charged situation when prompted by an adult

....

Middle school (grades 6-8)

_____ Able to walk away from confrontation or provocation by a peer

_____ Can say no to a fun activity if other plans have already been made

_____ Resists saying hurtful things when with a group of friends

....

If you gave your child mostly 2s or higher for each ability for her age, you can probably say your child is not seriously deficient in response inhibition but would benefit from some tweaking. If you gave the child all 0s or 1s, you probably need to teach the skill directly. To help you design your own intervention strategy, we provide a couple of fairly detailed scenarios depicting situations that parents frequently seek our help with. Following the description of an intervention we've used, we give you a template, or outline, that breaks the intervention down by the kinds of elements we discussed in the first half of the book. In each case, we describe environmental modifications, a skill instruction sequence, and an incentive to help reinforce the child for using the skills. Don't forget to use our suggestions in Chapter 3 for boosting your success with such interventions when you and your child have a weakness in response inhibition.

Building Response Inhibition in Everyday Situations

• *Always assume that the youngest children have very little impulse control.* This may seem like stating the obvious, but when you have a kid who's smart but scattered, emphasis on *smart*, it's remarkably easy to forget that native intelligence doesn't translate to response inhibition when the child in question is only 4, 5, or 6. Even though response inhibition starts to develop in infancy, preschool and primary-grade children have a lot of competing drives to contend with, whether it's the desire to have a four-scoop ice cream cone instead of a single scoop, to stay up late because he doesn't feel even a little bit tired, or to dart across the school parking lot to see his best friend when the lot is teeming with cars trying to get back on the road. Whether it's removing temptations like controlling snacks, establishing routines such as consistent bedtimes, making rules about behavior (such as displaying good table manners and sharing toys with a playmate), or providing close supervision in situations where impulses might get a child in trouble (such as in that busy parking lot), setting limits for our kids introduces the youngest kids to impulse control and thus encourages response inhibition.

- *Help your child learn to delay gratification by using formal waiting periods for things she wants to do or have.* Learning to wait for something is the foundation for the more sophisticated executive skills we want children to develop over time. If your child has trouble waiting, set a kitchen timer and let her know when the bell rings she can have or do what she's asked for. Make the time lag small initially and gradually increase the time delay. First/then schedules accomplish the same goal ("First do your spelling homework, then you get to play a video game").

- *Requiring children to earn some things they want is another way to teach them to delay gratification and inhibit impulses.* If this is hard for them, give them a visible means to mark their progress, such as a graph or sticker chart.

- Help children understand that there are consequences for poor impulse control. In some cases the consequences will be naturally occurring events (if your son keeps hitting his playmates, they will soon not want to play with him anymore), while in other cases you will need to impose consequences ("If you can't share the Xbox with your brother, I'll have to take it away for a while").

- *Prepare your child for situations that require impulse control by reviewing them in advance.* Ask, "What are the rules for playing video games?" or "What will you do if there's a long line of kids waiting to go down the biggest slide at the water park?"

- *Practice response inhibition in role-playing situations.* Kids, just like adults, may have more trouble controlling impulses than usual when the situation is emotionally charged or they're overtired or overstimulated (such as during holidays). In those cases in particular, pose a predictably dicey dilemma and play the role of someone who might challenge your child's ability to think before acting or speaking.

- *Cue your child before he enters a situation that calls for a specific behavior you're targeting and then reward him for exhibiting self-control.* Let's say you're working hard at helping your child avoid getting into fights when he goes outdoors to play with neighbors. Before your son goes outside, ask, "What behavior are we working on?" and then watch how things go so you can offer a reward quickly after your child shows that he's practicing self-control. It's important for you or the child's other parent to be right there (or at least able to watch from a short distance, such as through a window) so you can observe the behavior directly rather than relying on your child's report. Being present is also important because you need to be able to reinforce your child's positive behavior as it occurs.

- *See routine 16 in Chapter 10 for a general teaching sequence to help children learn to control impulsive behavior.*

A Parent's Fondest Dream: Reducing Interruptions during Phone Calls

Mekhi, an active 6-year-old, is the younger of two children in his family. He can play for short periods of time alone but likes it better if he has a friend to play with or one of his parents is available. His 9-year-old sister has little patience for the games he wants to play. His parents, particularly Mom, are especially frustrated by Mekhi's interrupting when they're on the phone or when someone comes to the door. For example, Mekhi might be looking at a book when the phone rings. As soon as his mother picks it up, Mekhi is there. Sometimes it might be a repeated question: "Mom, can you play a game with me?" Or he might be complaining about his sister being mean to him. Often he tugs on her arm, sits in her lap, or touches her face. Mekhi's father gets similar interruptions but is less bothered by them because he's not around as often and Mom gets the brunt of this behavior.

Mekhi's parents have tried a number of techniques to get around these disruptions. If the phone call is short, they alternate between ignoring Mekhi and telling him to be quiet. Once in a while, if the call is important, they will try to "buy" quiet behavior with the promise of a new toy. Sometimes they will put the call off until later. When Mekhi is particularly noisy, they threaten a consequence when they get off the phone. They haven't had much success with any approach and would like to see Mekhi begin to manage this behavior on his own.

Mekhi's parents ask Mekhi if he could help them solve a problem. They describe their problem and explain that it's important for them to be able to talk and listen to other people on the phone. They give a few examples, and Mekhi also gives an example of when he talks on the phone. His parents ask if Mekhi could think of something he could do instead of talking to them during phone calls. He suggests playing with trucks or watching TV. TV time is already limited to a certain part of the day, so the parents ask for another idea, and Mekhi chooses Legos. Mekhi makes a card with drawings of trucks and Legos and with help writes the words underneath each picture. They will keep the card by the phone, and when the phone rings or when Mom or Dad need to make a call, they will show it to Mekhi and he will choose one or the other activity. For the first few weeks his parents make "practice" phone calls or ask family or friends to call occasionally so Mekhi can practice his plan. They realize that in the early stages the calls need to be short. They also realize that they need to reinforce Mekhi's desirable behavior frequently (at least twice a minute) by telling him that he's doing a good job playing. Whenever they failed to do this in the first few days, Mekhi stopped playing and came to them. From this, they recognized that they had to praise him before he interrupted them. They make a deal with him that if he does a good job, he can pick out some new Legos or trucks to add to his collection.

Step 1: Establish Behavioral Goal

Target executive skill(s): Response inhibition

Specific behavioral objective: Engage in independent play and do not interrupt when parents are on the phone.

Step 2: Design Intervention

What environmental supports will be provided to help reach the target goal?

- Availability of preferred toys
- Picture card of play choices
- Parent cue to choose when phone rings

What specific skill will be taught, who will teach the skill, and what procedure will be used to teach it?

Skill: Response inhibition (learning to play independently instead of seeking out parents when they are on the phone)

Who will teach the skill? Parents

Procedure:

- Mekhi chooses two preferred play activities.
- Parents make up picture cards for these activities.
- When parents are going to phone or phone rings, they present card and Mekhi chooses one activity.
- Parents, during call, praise him for continuing to play.

What incentives will be used to help motivate the child to use/practice the skill?

- Parents praise Mekhi for playing.
- Parents add to Mekhi's toy collection for these activities if he does well.

👍 Keys to Success 👍

- *Don't wait to reinforce the behavior you're looking for.* Parents sometimes feel silly praising a child for sticking with the chosen activity when the child has been involved with it for only a minute. But as Mekhi's parents quickly discovered, if you wait, you're leaving a window wide open for your child to abandon the activity and come looking for attention, in which case the whole exercise has already gotten off on the wrong foot.

- *Don't assume that quick success means the problem has been solved.* In most cases, if you follow the plan and pay attention to your child at short intervals, you will see success quickly. It's then far too easy to get overconfident—or simply to forget to praise your child because you're not being interrupted. But if you abandon this exercise prematurely, the old behavior pattern is bound to return—

(cont.)

> and then you're likely to decide the plan simply failed. Attention must be faded gradually (for example, from every 30 seconds to every 45 or 60 and so on) until your child can engage in the activity for 5-10 minutes or more without interrupting. How long the child can stay with the activity is somewhat dependent on age, so with younger children (kindergarten to early elementary grades), you should continue to check in at least every few minutes.

Calling a Truce: Discouraging Fights with Siblings

Evan is a 13-year-old seventh grader. He's the type of boy who can't seem to let a comment from someone else pass without a reaction. He's quick and can be funny, but his sarcastic and other inappropriate comments have also gotten him into trouble.

Evan has two younger brothers, 10 and 7. He and his brothers have always had their conflicts, but the situation seems to have worsened over the past year, since Evan entered middle school. Like many older brothers his age, Evan finds his siblings annoying. Just having them around at times is irritating, but he feels they aggravate the issue with their "dumb" comments and by competing for TV and video game time and attention at dinner.

Evan feels that age has its privileges, and he would prefer that his brothers not speak unless spoken to. They obviously don't see it this way. His mother knows that sometimes his siblings just want his attention. She also feels that, as the oldest, Evan should be able to take the "high road" and better tolerate his brothers' comments and behavior. Not only has Evan been unable to do this, but he reacts quickly to any comment from his brothers, screaming and at times threatening them.

The situation has reached the point where whenever Evan and either one or both brothers are home they end up in a fight. Mother either ends up as the referee or disciplining Evan for his overreaction. She's had enough. While she understands that all the boys have a role in this, she also feels that if Evan is less reactive, she can better manage his brothers.

Mom approaches Evan to talk about the situation and to try to devise a plan. Evan admits he doesn't like fighting all the time, but he doesn't know how to keep himself from reacting. He feels he deserves some privacy and believes he could control himself better if he were not around his brothers as much. At the same time he hears what his mother is saying and is willing to spend some (a little) time with his brothers as long as it's controlled.

Evan and his mother agree that his room will be his private space, and his brothers cannot enter without his permission. Initially, he agrees he'll be available to do something with them for 20 minutes a day during the week and 30 minutes on weekend days. This does not count family time such as meals and planned family activities. Evan feels—and his mom agrees—that fights are less likely if the time is structured, so they get a list of preferred games and other activities from his brothers that they can pick from to play with Evan. He is willing to play whatever they select and says he will try not to argue about rules or correct them because this is their time. Evan gets to say when he is available or not by flipping a sign on his door that says *available* on one side and *not available* on the other.

Evan's quick verbal reactions are a little trickier to manage. Mom first agrees that if she hears one of the boys say something provocative (teasing, insults, etc.), she will discipline him. However, she will not accept third-party reports from Evan or his brothers. Beyond that, she believes that Evan will need reminders and some incentive to help him control this behavior. He has wanted a cell phone, and although his mother has thought privately about getting him one, she has not acted on or promised this. She proposes that when Evan is not in his room, for each 2 hours he goes without reacting to and fighting with his brothers, she will give him a point. She figures that he can earn 2–3 points per day and more on weekends.

Mom tells Evan that she will remind him of the deal each day. If partway through the 2 hours he fights with his brothers, she will reset the clock. As soon as Evan reaches 100 points, she agrees to buy the phone, and then he'll earn minutes with his points. Although this system requires a fair amount of monitoring by Mom, it's a small price to pay for eliminating the disruption the fighting causes. At home, Evan gets in the habit of ignoring his brothers' comments, and he actually enjoys some of the time they play together. His mother is happy because she sees a decrease in fighting. After about 5 weeks, she is able to use a more informal approach for Evan to earn his phone minutes. She and Evan rate how the day went just before bed. If they both agree it went *great*, then he earns the maximum number of minutes. If they agree it went *OK*, he earns a lower number of minutes, and if they decide it went *terrible*, then no minutes are earned. If they find they disagree on the ratings, they move back to the more formal point system.

Step 1: Establish Behavioral Goal

Target executive skill(s): Response inhibition

Specific behavioral objective: Refrain from threatening comments in response to comments from brothers

Step 2: Design Intervention

What environmental supports will be provided to help reach the target goal?
- Private space and time
- Mother will referee brothers' comments to Evan
- Structured activities and limited time for brothers' interactions

(cont.)

What specific skill will be taught, who will teach the skill, and what procedure will be used to teach it?

Skill: Response inhibition (indicating availability to brothers and controlling his reaction to his brothers' comments)

Who will teach the skill? Mother

Procedure:

- Evan designates when he is and is not available.
- He agrees to time-limited structured play activities with brothers.
- Mother maintains boundaries and manages unacceptable comments from brothers.
- Mother cues Evan daily about inhibiting reaction to brothers.
- Evan leaves situation and goes to room if frustrated.

What incentives will be used to help motivate the child to use/practice the skill?

- Evan is guaranteed private time and space for himself.
- Evan can earn a cell phone and usage time on an ongoing basis.

👍 Keys to Success 👍

- *Consistency is critical right from the start.* Evan needs to see that his mother is making an effort to discipline his younger brothers when they say or do something to annoy him. If this doesn't happen, he'll see the system as unfair and revert to his old reactions. If you're not quick to manage younger siblings' behavior in an intervention like this, seeing their comments as "no big deal" and expecting your older child to ignore them, the plan will break down.

- *Anticipate some fighting to continue since you won't see everything that goes on between siblings.* Evan's mother refused to take reports on behaviors she did not witness, which makes sense. But that means there *will* be behavior she doesn't witness. If this becomes a problem, you may need to set a rule that if an argument starts, the boys go to their respective rooms for at least 15 minutes.

- *If the plan doesn't seem to be working, it could be because you've allotted too long a time for the children to play together at first.* Twenty minutes may initially be too long for Evan to play with his brothers, in which case a shorter, successful playtime can be built on over time.

- *Follow-through is essential when you agree to pay a child for the desired behavior.* "Paying" Evan for not arguing/fighting was effective only because his mother took great care to fulfill her promise to give him the points he had earned and then bought him a phone promptly once he'd earned 100 points.

12

Enhancing Working Memory

Working memory is the capacity to hold information in mind while performing complex tasks. We rely on working memory all the time. It's the ability to run out to the store to buy a few things and remember what they are without having to write them down. When you remember to stop by the dry cleaner on your way home from work, you're using working memory. When you look up a phone number in the phone book and remember it long enough to make the call, you're using working memory. When your spouse asks you to do something and you say, "I'll do it as soon as I finish loading the dishwasher," and then you actually remember to do it, chances are your working memory is pretty good. Odds are it's not so good, however, if you can't remember anyone's birthday, you tend to return home with only half your errands done unless you have a written agenda, and you'll do anything to avoid having to introduce people at a cocktail party because you can't remember anyone's name. In that case, be sure to use the tips in Chapter 3 to help you enhance your child's working memory when you have the same weakness.

How Working Memory Develops

Working memory begins to develop fairly early in infancy. When you're playing with a baby and you hide a favorite toy under a blanket, you know the baby is using working memory if he lifts the blanket to retrieve the toy. This is because the baby is able to hold an image of the toy in mind as well as the memory of what you did to hide it.

Children develop *nonverbal* working memory before they develop *verbal* working memory because this skill begins to emerge before language does. When children develop language, however, their working memory skills expand, because now they can draw on visual imagery and language to retrieve information.

As we told you in Chapter 1, when children and teenagers perform tasks that require executive skills such as working memory, they rely on the prefrontal cortex to do all the work rather than distributing the workload to other specialized regions of the brain, as adults are able to do. Thus, activating working memory takes more conscious effort with children and with teenagers than it does with adults, which may help explain why they are less inclined to use their working memory to complete daily routine tasks.

We tend naturally to limit our expectations for working memory in very young children. Before the age of 3, we generally expect children to remember only things that are in close proximity—either in time or in space. If we want them to do something, we don't say, "Would you mind putting your toys away after you finish watching *Barney*?" (unless we also expect to cue them once *Barney* is over). And while we might ask them to put all their blocks in the toy box while we're standing in the playroom with them, we generally don't instruct them to go to their bedroom and do a similar task all by themselves.

Gradually, we're able to stretch both time and distance in terms of what we expect our children to be able to remember. In the questionnaire below, you can evaluate where your child might fall on the developmental ladder, based on the kinds of tasks children are capable of carrying out independently at various childhood stages. Using this scale will give you a closer look than the scales in Chapter 2 did at how well your child uses the skill of working memory.

HOW GOOD IS YOUR CHILD'S WORKING MEMORY?

Use the following scale to rate how well your child performs each of the tasks listed. At each level, children can be expected to perform all the tasks listed fairly well to very well.

Scale

0—Never or rarely

1—Does but not well (about 25% of the time)

2—Does fairly well (about 75% of the time)

3—Does very well (always or almost always)

Preschool/kindergarten

_____ Runs simple errands (e.g., gets shoes from bedroom when asked)

_____ Remembers instructions that were just given

_____ Follows a routine with only one prompt per step (e.g., brushing teeth after breakfast)

Lower elementary (grades 1-3)

____ Able to run an errand with two to three steps

____ Remembers instructions that were given a couple of minutes earlier

____ Follows two steps of a routine with one prompt

Upper elementary (grades 4-5)

____ Remembers to perform a routine chore after school without reminder

____ Takes books, papers, assignments to and from school

____ Keeps track of changing daily schedule (e.g., different activities after school)

Middle school (grades 6-8)

____ Able to keep track of assignments and classroom expectations of multiple teachers

____ Remembers events or responsibilities that deviate from the norm (e.g., permission slips for field trips, special instructions regarding extracurricular activities, etc.)

____ Remembers multistep directions, given sufficient time or practice

From *Smart but Scattered* by Peg Dawson and Richard Guare. Copyright 2009 by The Guilford Press.

Building Working Memory in Everyday Situations

• *Make eye contact with your child before telling him something you want him to remember.*

• *Keep external distractions to a minimum if you want your child's full attention* (for example, turn off the television or turn down the volume).

• *Have the child repeat back to you what you just said so you know she has heard you.*

• *Use written reminders*—picture schedules, lists, and schedules, depending on the age of the child. Prompt the child at each step to "check your schedule" or "look at your list."

• *Rehearse with the child what you expect him to remember just before the situation* (for example, "What do you need to say to Aunt Mary after she gives you your birthday present?").

• *Help the child think about ways to help her remember something important that she thinks will work for her.*

• With children in middle school, use cell phones, text messages, or instant messages (IMs) to remind them of important things they have to do.

• *Consider using a reward for remembering key information or imposing a penalty for forgetting.* For example, a child might be allowed to rent a video game on the weekend if he goes a whole week without forgetting to bring home all his homework materials. Rewards and penalties are useful when your child's working memory is only mildly underdeveloped.

Ending the Waiting Game: Teaching Your Child to Get Dressed without Dawdling

Annie is a bright 8-year-old second grader who can be absent-minded at times but is one of the more advanced students in her class. She has a variety of interests and is a good friend to her peers. Her mother would like to see her develop more independence, particularly around recurring tasks such as picking out clothes and getting dressed for school. Because Annie's best friend, Sarah, has been managing the dressing process for the better part of a year, Mrs. Smith doesn't think this is an unrealistic expectation for Annie. She and Annie have talked about it, and Annie has said she'd like to do it, particularly because she'd like to choose her own clothes.

However, each morning a familiar pattern unfolds: "Annie, it's time to start getting dressed." "OK, Mom, " Annie says as she heads upstairs. Mom busies herself getting ready for work and after about 10 minutes calls to Annie. "Annie, how's it coming?" "OK, Mom," comes the reply. After another 5 minutes, Mom calls out, "Annie, you need to move it along." "OK," comes the reply again. Shortly after that Mom goes upstairs to find Annie sitting on the floor drawing, still in her pajamas. "Annie!" says Mom with great frustration while grabbing some clothes. Annie begins to protest the choices, but her mom silences her and stays long enough to see that Annie is well into getting dressed before telling her to be downstairs "in one minute!"

In a calmer moment, Annie and her mother talk it over and decide that Mom will watch Annie go through this task to decide what might help. Although a bit slow, Annie is able to pick out her clothes and get dressed without major problems. However, in spite of her good intentions, when Annie tries to manage the task on her own, her mother still ends up frustrated at having to give Annie repeated reminders.

They decide to try another approach. If Annie agrees to work with her on a plan, Mom agrees to let Annie pick out some clothes she has wanted. First, they make a list of the steps in the dressing process and Annie writes these down. Annie says that sometimes it's hard for her to choose what to wear, so they decide to put out a choice of two outfits the night before and Annie picks out a place where they will be kept. They then do a pretend walk-through and Mom takes a digital photo of each step. Annie matches the steps she wrote to the pictures and hangs the "picture board" next to her closet.

In the beginning, Annie thinks that besides cueing her that it's time to get dressed, it would help if Mom came upstairs with her to watch her get started and then left. Mother reluctantly agrees, provided this is temporary. The final issue is time. Morning is usually rushed, and when Annie is slow, her mother gets upset. They buy an inexpensive digital timer, and Annie feels like 12 to 15 minutes is plenty of time to finish. Mom agrees. Because Annie sometimes gets lost in the process, she sets the timer for 5-minute intervals; that way, even if she gets involved with something else, the timer can be a cue. As an added check, when her mother hears the timer, she yells to Annie, "What step?" and Annie says where she is in the sequence.

Over the first few weeks, Annie has one or two mornings where Mom has to prod her, but overall they're both pleased. Annie feels comfortable with Mom not going upstairs, but she still likes the verbal check-ins and the praise from Mom when she does a good job. They also plan a shopping trip together.

Step 1: Establish Behavioral Goal

Target executive skill(s): Working memory

Specific behavioral objective: Annie will complete her morning dressing routine within 15 minutes with no more than one adult prompt

Step 2: Design Intervention

What environmental supports will be provided to help reach the target goal?

- Advance selection of clothes
- Timer
- Parent observation and prompts in early stages of the plan

What specific skill will be taught, who will teach the skill, and what procedure will be used to teach it?

Skill: Working memory (follow a daily morning routine)

Who will teach skill? Mother

Procedure:

- Mother and Annie meet to discuss the problem and desired outcome.
- They make a list of steps and Annie writes them.
- Two outfits are selected the night before.
- Annie does a walk-through, and Mom takes a picture of each step.
- Annie matches the written steps to the pictures and posts the sequence next to her closet.

(cont.)

- Annie decides the time needed and they get a timer.
- Mom agrees to cue her and watch her start for a week or so.
- Mom checks in when the timer beeps at each 5-minute interval.
- Mom keeps track of the number of reminders needed each day.

What incentives will be used to help motivate the child to use/practice the skill?

- Praise from mother
- Purchase new clothes

👍 Keys to Success 👍

- *Be enthusiastic and thorough in the early stages.* This system is usually successful when first implemented because it's novel and provides systematic cueing as well as an incentive. When it breaks down, it's often because parents haven't monitored the system closely enough in the initial stages.
- *Err on the side of cueing for too long.* In our experience, many kids need ongoing cueing, and when parents are reluctant to provide it initial gains often disappear. If your child "relapses" when you start to pull back on cueing, step it up and fade out of this role very gradually, in baby steps.

The Absent-Minded Athlete: Teaching Your Child to Keep Track of Sports Equipment

It's 7:30 Monday morning, and Jake, a 14-year-old eighth grader, is in front of the family computer instant messaging (IMing) his friends. Because he is dressed, has eaten, and says his stuff (school backpack and soccer bag) is ready, his dad is okay with him being on the computer until the bus comes at 7:45. He has a soccer game today, and to be on the safe side, Dad says, "Jake, check your soccer bag to make sure you have everything." "No problem," comes the reply as he continues to IM with his friends. A couple of minutes before the bus comes his father cues Jake and his sister to get ready. When Jake comes into the hall, his father asks if he has checked his soccer stuff, and he quickly opens the bag and rummages through it. "What did you do with my shin guards?" he accuses his father in a panic. Irritated and unable to resist the urge, Dad replies that he wore them to work. Jake, frustrated, says, "My coach will kill me, and I won't be able to play." The bus arrives, and Dad tells him they'll try to work something out, although he's not sure what. At the game his coach is upset with him and tells him that he can't play. Just before the game starts, his father meets a parent who has an extra pair of shin guards. He debates whether to let Jake suffer the consequences of not playing, but because this has happened before and it hasn't solved the problem, he doesn't want to see him in more trouble with his coach. He gives the guards to his son, but they agree that this will not happen again.

That night they talk about a system to help Jake organize and remember equipment. Because he is a three-sport athlete, this is basically a year-round problem. Dad suggests a list that he can use to check off equipment as he packs his bag. While this might help him know if he has what he needs in his bag, it doesn't solve the problem of organizing his equipment so that when he needs it it will be readily available. His father jokes that maybe he should just sleep with his equipment on the night before a game so he can just pack it in the morning and know he has everything. Jake says that maybe they should make a cutout of him and hang the equipment on the cutout. This would give him a place to store his equipment and easily see what's missing. They agree to put labels on the cutout for each piece of equipment needed, and Dad agrees to cue Jake the night before to check the cutout and pack. For his part, Jake agrees that when Dad cues him to do this the night before, he will do it and not wait until the morning. They also agree that if he doesn't follow through and forgets something, Dad won't rescue him. They make the cutout, and Jake labels it for the current soccer season. He makes hooks to hang things and tries it out by putting all the equipment on the cutout while his father watches. They are satisfied that the cutout will work.

Step 1: Establish Behavioral Goal

Target executive skill(s): Working memory

Specific behavioral objective: Jake will organize his sports equipment before each game and have the equipment he needs for each game with no more than one adult prompt

Step 2: Design Intervention

What environmental supports will be provided to help reach the target goal?

- A cutout of Jake that will be labeled with equipment needed for practice and games.
- Reminder from his dad the night before a game to check and pack his equipment.

What specific skill will be taught, who will teach the skill, and what procedure will be used to teach it?

Skill: Working memory (remember all required sports equipment for practice and games)

(cont.)

Who will teach the skill? Father

Procedure:

- Jake and Dad meet and agree on a plan for organizing the equipment.
- Jake, with Dad's help, makes a cutout.
- Jake makes labels and hooks for all equipment and puts them on the cutout.
- He tries one practice run with his father watching.
- Dad agrees to cue him to get equipment ready the night before.
- For two weeks, Dad checks with him after he has given the cue to ensure that he has followed through.

What incentives will be used to help motivate the child to use/practice the skill?

- Jake will be able to participate in sports without experiencing consequences from coaches for not having equipment.

👍 Keys to Success 👍

- *Don't rely on your child's statement that he or she has acted on your cue.* In this example the cutout served as a reminder and an organizing tool for Jake. While this may be enough in most cases, children with working memory weaknesses, when asked about or cued to remember something, will often indicate that they have done what they need to do or will take care of it and then proceed to forget. Therefore you'll need to follow up the cue with a check to see if your child has in fact acted on the cue. Acting at the time that the cue is given is key, which may involve your checking on a more frequent basis until the desired behavior is established.

13

Improving Emotional Control

Emotional control is the ability to manage emotions to achieve goals, complete tasks, or control and direct your behavior. If this is a strength for you, you're not only able to handle the daily ups and downs of life easily but can maintain your cool in more emotionally charged situations as well—whether it's a confrontation with a hot-tempered boss or with a teenage son challenging parental authority. Having the skill to control your emotions means not only being able to control your temper but also being able to manage unpleasant feelings such as anxiety, frustration, and disappointment. Being able to control your emotions also means being able to tap into positive emotions to help you overcome obstacles or to keep you going during difficult times. It's not hard to see how important this skill can be to success during childhood and beyond.

Some of us demonstrate the skill in some settings but not in others. Most of us, kids and adults alike, have a "public self" and a "private self," and different rules seem to govern each of these personas. Does your child hold it together at school but then fall apart at home? Do you keep your cool at work but let your guard down with your family? This shift isn't uncommon, and it's not always a problem. But it can be. If either you or your child finds controlling your emotions such a strain that you can't make the effort once you're within the confines of home and family, feelings are likely to get hurt or chronic tension may be chipping away at your family. In that case explosions over the kinds of tasks that your child struggles with due to executive skill deficits may be a major problem for you. That's an indication that boosting emotional control is a priority for you and/or your child. In fact, if you both struggle to maintain emotional control, you'll want to take advantage of the tips in Chapter 3 to give yourselves the best chance at success with the interventions you design based on this chapter. If taking an objective look at the situation tells you that a lack of emotional control on your part is contributing to your child's problem, you might consider consulting a therapist for help.

How Emotional Control Develops

In early infancy, babies expect parents to respond to their physical needs (food, bottle, diaper change) as they arise, and when these needs are met consistently and predictably, babies are generally able to hold their emotions within bounds. Of course there are always times when adults can't supply immediate relief, so babies gradually learn to soothe themselves. There are some exceptions to this typical developmental progression—colicky babies might be best described as infants with weak ability to regulate their responses—but most infants seem to outgrow this phase and learn self-soothing techniques just like other babies.

In toddlerhood and the preschool years, however, you can begin to see individual variations in emotional regulation abilities. Some little kids go through the "terrible twos" with only mild tantrums, while others have emotional meltdowns whose frequency or intensity challenges even the most unflappable parents. At around age 3, most children develop rituals, such as a precise sequence of steps they expect to happen every night at bedtime. Despite these expectations, you'll notice that some children can roll with changes in the routine while others get very agitated if the sequence is disrupted in any way. Kids with low emotional control can therefore appear to be very rigid. If your child fits this description, you might benefit from reading Chapter 19 too; there's a lot of overlap between the emotional control and flexibility skills.

In elementary school, children whose ability to manage their emotions is weak frequently encounter social problems; they may have trouble sharing toys, losing at games or sports, or not getting their way during make-believe games with friends. Kids who have good emotional control are the ones you'll notice can make compromises, accept winning and losing at games with equanimity, and may act as peacemakers in altercations between peers.

Adolescence brings new challenges for emotional control as it does for many other executive skills. This age group as a whole is more susceptible to breakdowns in the ability to handle stress. Teenagers rely on the prefrontal cortex to tell the rest of the brain how to behave. In times of stress, in the words of one brain researcher, "they are using up prefrontal cortex like crazy." This means the part of the brain responsible for managing executive skills becomes overloaded as teenagers try to inhibit responses (see Chapter 11), tap into working memory (Chapter 12), and control their emotions all at the same time. No wonder teenagers often make slow or bad decisions or, worse, bad *fast* decisions. Teens who lag behind in developing emotional control will be at an even bigger disadvantage, experiencing more than their share of emotional turmoil during a phase of development that's marked by emotional ups and downs.

Knowing this, you would do well to protect your middle schooler by doing whatever you can to minimize the stress that leads to bad decisions. Meanwhile, you can also help him boost his emotional control using the strategies in this chapter. It's well worth the effort: teenagers who can manage their emotions are less likely to argue with teachers or coaches, can handle performance situations (games, exams) without excessive anxiety, and can bounce back quickly from disappointment.

HOW WELL DOES YOUR CHILD REGULATE EMOTIONS?

Use the following scale to rate how well your child performs each of the tasks listed. At each level, children can be expected to perform all the tasks listed fairly well to very well.

Scale

0—Never or rarely

1—Does but not well (about 25% of the time)

2—Does fairly well (about 75% of the time)

3—Does very well (always or almost always)

Preschool/kindergarten

_____ Can recover fairly quickly from a disappointment or a change in plans

_____ Can use nonphysical solutions when another child takes a toy he or she was playing with

_____ Can play in a group without becoming overly excited

Lower elementary (grades 1-3)

_____ Can tolerate criticism from an adult (e.g., a teacher reprimand)

_____ Can deal with perceived "unfairness" without becoming overly upset

_____ Can adjust behavior quickly depending on the situation (e.g., calming down after recess)

Upper elementary (grades 4-5)

_____ Doesn't overreact to losing a game or not being selected for an award

_____ Can accept not getting what he or she wants when working or playing in a group

_____ Acts with restraint in response to teasing

Middle school (grades 6-8)

_____ Can "read" reactions from friends and adjust behavior accordingly

_____ Can anticipate outcomes and prepare for possible disappointment

_____ Can be appropriately assertive (e.g., asking teacher for help, inviting someone to dance at a school dance)

Improving Emotional Control
in Everyday Situations

- *With younger children, regulate the environment.* You can reduce the likelihood that the child's emotions will get out of control by building in routines, particularly around mealtimes, naptimes, and bedtimes. Avoid placing the child in situations where she is likely to become overstimulated or find ways to remove her quickly from those situations when you sense she's beginning to lose control.

- *Prepare your child by talking with him about what to expect and what he can do if he starts to feel overwhelmed.* Some problem situations are simply unavoidable but can be defused with a little advance work.

- *Give your child coping strategies.* What options for escape can you provide? Younger kids may be able to come to an agreement with the teacher or other supervising adult about a signal that means the child needs a break. At home, you and your child might agree that when things get too hot to handle, the child can say something like "I need to go to my bedroom for a few minutes to be alone" to tell you a break is needed. Simple self-soothing strategies can include picking up and holding a favorite stuffed animal (for a younger child) or plugging into soothing music on an iPod (for an older child). Or have your child learn relaxation techniques, such as deep breathing and progressive relaxation, which involves alternately tensing and relaxing the major muscle groups in the body. Type "relaxation for kids" into a search engine to find resources that will provide instructions for these techniques.

- *Give your child a script to follow for problem situations.* This doesn't have to be complicated, just something short she can say to herself to help her manage her emotions. It's helpful to model these kinds of self-statements. For instance, if your child gives up without trying when a homework assignment appears difficult, you might say to her, "Here's what I want you to say to yourself before starting this: *I know this will be hard for me, but I'm going to keep trying. If I get stuck after trying hard, I will ask for help.*" Children with weak emotional control are more prone than peers to dissolve in tears or throw a tantrum when forced to stick with tasks they find frustrating or difficult.

- *Read stories in which characters exhibit the behaviors you want your child to learn.* *The Little Engine That Could* is a good example of one that models the positive emotions (in this case, the determination represented by "I think I can, I think I can") that kids with weak emotional control often have trouble accessing. Children's librarians may be a good resource to consult.

- If these efforts don't alleviate the problem, you may want to work with a counselor or therapist trained in cognitive behavioral therapy. We also recommend two books that explain this approach within the context of specific emotional control problems: *What to Do When You Worry Too Much* and *What to Do When You Grumble Too Much*, both written by Dawn Huebner. They are written for children and parents to read together and include exercises children can do to help them understand the problem and develop coping strategies.

Smart and Showing It: Beating Test Anxiety

Courtney is a 14-year-old eighth grader. She has always been a very responsible girl, the oldest of three children in her family, and her parents expect her to do well. Courtney plays field hockey and has a small group of close friends she has known since elementary school. She is a B student and has to put in a fair amount of effort for the grades she gets. Math, in particular, can be a struggle, especially this year with prealgebra.

Courtney has a major test coming up in math and is a wreck just thinking about it. She has really studied the material and gone over the problems she didn't understand with one of her friends. She feels like she understands the material now, but this hasn't decreased her worry about not doing well on the test. Her mother sees that Courtney is on edge, but Courtney says she is "just tired." She feels like if she tells her parents she's worried, they will just focus on how important it is to do well and this will only make her more anxious. Courtney doesn't sleep well the night before the test, and her stomach is churning when she gets to class. She is able to answer the first few questions but then "blanks" on two major problems. Courtney does what she can, and while relieved that the test is over, she knows she didn't do well. Her fears are confirmed when she gets her test grade, a D, and she is frustrated because she realizes she knew how to do the problems but just panicked. She tells her parents, and they blow up. Her father says, "If this happens in high school, you can forget about college if you get grades like that." Courtney breaks down, telling her parents how hard she worked and how she "froze" when it came to the test. Seeing her reaction, her parents realize that demanding she do better will probably only make the situation more stressful for her.

Together, Courtney and her parents work out a plan. Because not all demands lead to major worry, they discuss how to tell when her worries reach a point that they hurt her performance. Courtney suggests she use a scale of 1 to 10, then she decides it will be a problem if her anxious feelings get above 4. In that case, Courtney says, it would help her if she could tell her parents something is bothering her. But it won't help if they stress about it or offer their standard solution, "You need to study more!" Her parents agree to listen, ask if there is some way they can help, and try not to stress. If they act otherwise, they suggest that Courtney remind them of their role, and she agrees to this.

From past experience, her parents know that Courtney's worry about performance demands decreases if she has a plan beforehand, so they discuss this with her. Courtney agrees and proposes the following plan to handle her anxiety about tests:

- For any subject she is worried about, she will meet with the teacher prior to any tests, explain that she sometimes gets anxious about tests, and ask if the teacher recommends any specific study techniques to help her master the material.

- If, as with math, she has ongoing difficulty, she will try to set up a schedule to review material with the teacher regularly.
- She will meet with her counselor to see if she has any strategies to manage stress and worrying.

Her parents think this is a very good plan, and they are impressed with Courtney's thoughtfulness and problem solving. For the next math test Courtney follows the plan. Her parents are more relaxed, which in turn helps Courtney. She is more comfortable taking the test, although a little disappointed with her grade, a C+. But her teacher, seeing her effort, offers the option of extra credit.

Step 1: Establish Behavioral Goal

Target executive skill(s): Emotional control

Specific behavioral objective: Courtney will improve her performance on tests to Cs or higher

Step 2: Design Intervention

What environmental supports will be provided to help reach the target goal?

- Scale to measure anxiety
- Nonjudgmental support from parents
- Teacher assistance with studying
- Guidance support with test anxiety strategies

What specific skill will be taught, who will teach the skill, and what procedure will be used to teach it?

Skill: Emotional control (reduction of anxiety)

Who will teach the skill? Teachers, guidance counselor, Courtney

Procedure:

- Courtney will meet with teachers to learn specific study strategies.
- For her most difficult subjects, she will meet on a regular basis with teachers.
- She will meet with her guidance counselor for stress management strategies.

What incentives will be used to help motivate the child to use/practice the skill?

- Improved grades
- Reduced anxiety

👍 Keys to Success 👍

- *Be supportive, but otherwise refrain from offering your opinions unless you have some expertise in test anxiety.* Stick to listening and providing whatever help your child asks for. Going beyond that and giving advice about what she should do will likely only add to the pressure an anxious child already feels and be counter-productive.

- *Get whatever concrete help is available from teachers, the school psychologist, and any other professionals you may need to consult.* Courtney found it helpful when her teachers were available and could provide encouragement and offer concrete study tips. A school counselor/psychologist should also have some help-ful strategies and be able to work through them with a child suffering from test anxiety. If your child reports that the school counselor has not been able to help, ask your pediatrician to refer you to someone your child can could work with on a short-term basis to learn such strategies.

Staying in the Game:
How to Discourage Poor Sportsmanship

Mike is an active 7-year-old in second grade, the youngest in a family of three. Since he was a toddler, Mike has liked physical activities, especially sports, and he is clearly talented for a boy his age. He's excited about being able to play on "real" teams now and looks forward to games. At home when he has free time, Mike wants his parents or siblings to play and practice with him. However, with his family and with his teams, Mike expects to do well. When he or his team doesn't perform the way he expects, he can explode, complaining loudly, crying, and sometimes throw-ing equipment. When this happens, his coach sits him out or his parents remove him. After a time he settles down, but this action hasn't eliminated the behavior altogether; it still happens often enough to be a major concern to his parents. They've discussed stopping all sports participation but are reluctant to take this step because playing is so important to Mike. At the same time they realize they won't have any choice if Mike can't learn to tolerate errors and losing as part of sports.

After talking the situation over with one of the coaches and with friends who have two young sons involved in sports, they decide on a plan. They first sit down with Mike and explain that if he is to continue to play sports, they need to work out a way to help him change his behavior. Although he doesn't want to admit there's a problem, he agrees to a plan because he doesn't want to give up sports. The plan includes the following:

- *When he's upset about his own performance, Mike can express his frustration using agreed-on behaviors.* These include clenching his fists, crossing his arms and squeez-ing, and repeating a phrase of his choosing over and over quietly. If the frustration involves his team or a teammate, any public comment must be encouraging (for example, "Good try," "It's OK," etc.).

• *Together Mike and his parents write out scenarios for a few different situations that have happened,* substituting the use of his new strategies for his old behaviors.

• *Mike and his parents role-play what will happen by actually having him make a "mistake"* such as missing a basket or dropping a ball and then use one of his new strategies. They coach him through this and praise him for use of the strategy.

• *Before each game or practice, one of his parents reviews the rules and strategies with Mike and has him say how he will handle a frustrating situation if it comes up.* At the end of the game/practice Mike and his parents go over how he has done. If he's had no outbursts, he earns points toward eventually going to see one of his favorite professional teams play.

• *Mike agrees to try not to tantrum, scream, use disrespectful language, or throw things if he gets frustrated.* Any of these behaviors will result in his immediately leaving the game/practice and then missing the next one scheduled.

Mike is not completely successful in his first few weeks of games and practice, but his coach and parents note a major reduction in his outbursts and are confident that they're on the right track.

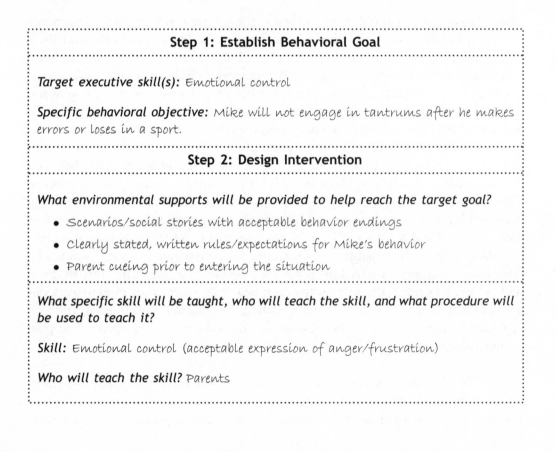

Step 1: Establish Behavioral Goal

Target executive skill(s): Emotional control

Specific behavioral objective: Mike will not engage in tantrums after he makes errors or loses in a sport.

Step 2: Design Intervention

What environmental supports will be provided to help reach the target goal?
• Scenarios/social stories with acceptable behavior endings
• Clearly stated, written rules/expectations for Mike's behavior
• Parent cueing prior to entering the situation

What specific skill will be taught, who will teach the skill, and what procedure will be used to teach it?

Skill: Emotional control (acceptable expression of anger/frustration)

Who will teach the skill? Parents

Procedure:

- Mike, together with his parents, will read scenarios of successful outcomes for typical problem situations.
- Mike and his parents will role-play the situation and use of a new strategy.
- Mike and his parents will review behavioral expectations/rules prior to the game.
- Mike and his parents will do a postgame review of his performance.
- Mike loses a practice or game for engaging in problem behavior.

What incentives will be used to help motivate the child to use/practice the skill?

- Mike is allowed to continue playing sports.

👍 Keys to Success 👍

Stick scrupulously to the game plan. This strategy's success depends on consistently following these steps:

1. Give the child an acceptable way to express his frustration.
2. Identify, with him, the situations where the behavior is most likely to occur.
3. Rehearse (role-play) the situation and cue the child on the appropriate behavior.
4. Cue him about your expectations just prior to entering the situation.
5. Remove him from the situation if necessary.

Skipping any one of these steps leaves the child vulnerable to losing control again since it's so hard for young children to "think on their feet" in frustrating situations.

14

Strengthening Sustained Attention

Sustained attention is the capacity to keep paying attention to a situation or task in spite of distractions, fatigue, or boredom. For us adults, this means sticking with tasks at work or chores at home by screening out distractions whenever possible and getting back to work as soon as feasible when interruptions are unavoidable. If your ability to sustain attention is weak, you'll find yourself jumping from task to task, often failing to finish the first before beginning the second. You might look for excuses to stop working, such as checking your email every 5 minutes or suddenly remembering a phone call you need to make. If you think you lack this skill, your efforts to help your child develop it will benefit from the tips in Chapter 3.

How the Skill of Sustaining Attention Develops

Picture a very young child at the beach. Isn't it amazing that the simple act of dropping a pebble into the water or building a canal can be a source of endless fun? Hands-on activities that would quickly bore us (or their babysitters, older siblings, or grandparents) to death may enthrall your young son or daughter for a long time. In fact children's ability to sustain attention when very little depends completely on how much interest they have in the activity. Very young children can stick with tasks for a long time if the activity appeals to them.

From the perspective of executive skills, however, sustaining attention is a challenge when the activity is something the child considers uninteresting or difficult, such as chores, schoolwork or homework, or sitting through lengthy adult-oriented events such as weddings or religious services. That we don't expect young children to sustain attention long in these kinds of situations is why many houses of worship will have children attend only the first 10 minutes or so of a service before sending them off to a religion-related activity outside the worship area. It's also why teachers' organizations, such as the American Federation of Teachers, recommend that children spend on homework no more than 10 minutes per grade level (10 minutes a night for first graders, 20 minutes a night for second graders, etc.). Good classroom teachers don't expect children to sit for long periods of time at their desks doing seatwork either, and skilled parents assign chores to younger children that can either be done quickly or be broken down into segments.

By the time children reach high school, they are expected to pay attention for longer periods of time in school and complete anywhere from 1 to 3 hours of homework a night. When schools made the switch to block scheduling a few years ago (longer classes that meet either for half the year or fewer times per week), it took teachers awhile to modify their teaching style so that lectures were no longer the primary instructional method. Even teenagers have a hard time focusing on a 90-minute lecture.

HOW WELL CAN YOUR CHILD SUSTAIN ATTENTION?

Use the following scale to rate how well your child performs each of the tasks listed. At each level, children can be expected to perform all the tasks listed fairly well to very well.

Scale

0—Never or rarely

1—Does but not well (about 25% of the time)

2—Does fairly well (about 75% of the time)

3—Does very well (always or almost always)

Preschool/kindergarten

_____ Can complete a 5-minute chore (may need supervision)

_____ Can sit through a preschool "circle time" (15-20 minutes)

_____ Can listen to one to two picture books at a sitting

Lower elementary (grades 1-3)

_____ Can spend 20-30 minutes on homework assignments

_____ Can complete a chore that takes 15-20 minutes

_____ Can sit through a meal of normal duration

(cont.)

Upper elementary (grades 4-5)

_____ Can spend 30-60 minutes on homework assignments

_____ Can complete chores that take 30-60 minutes (may need a break)

_____ Can attend to sports practice, church service, etc. for 60-90 minutes

Middle school (grades 6-8)

_____ Can spend 60-90 minutes on homework (may need one or more breaks)

_____ Can tolerate family commitments without complaining of boredom or getting into trouble

_____ Can complete chores that take up to 2 hours (may need breaks)

Strengthening Sustained Attention in Everyday Situations

• *Provide supervision.* Children can work longer when someone is with them, either offering encouragement or reminding them to stay on task. Maybe you can do some reading or paperwork of your own while your child is doing homework so that you're available to help your child stay on task while still spending the time productively.

• *Make increasing attention a gradual process.* Take a baseline by clocking how long your child can stick with a chore, homework, or other assigned task before needing a break. Once you establish the "base rate," set a kitchen timer for 2–3 minutes longer than the base rate and challenge your child to keep working until the timer rings.

• *Use a device that provides a visual depiction of elapsed time.* These devices can be bought from Time Timer (*www.timetimer.com*) in clock or wristwatch form as well as a software version.

• *Use a self-monitoring audiotape,* available at A.D.D. Warehouse (see the Resources), to help your child stay on task. This tape sounds electronic tones at random intervals. When the tone sounds, the child is to ask herself, "Was I paying attention?"

• *Make the task interesting.* Turn it into a challenge, a game, or a contest.

• *Use incentive systems.* Rewards should be powerful, frequent, and varied. For instance, you might award points for completed work or for work completed within specific time parameters.

- *Give your child something he can look forward to doing as soon as the task is finished.* Alternate between preferred and nonpreferred activities.
- *Offer praise for staying on-task.* Instead of focusing on your child when she is off-task (by nagging or reminding her to get back to work), provide attention and praise when your child is on-task.

Delicate Negotiations:
Reducing Distractions during Homework

Andy is a seventh grader with a busy life. He plays soccer on his school team and a travel team. In addition, he has started to play bass guitar with some friends and eventually would like to have a band.

Andy would like to get good grades, but compared to his other activities, most of his homework assignments seem very boring. He's pretty much set aside time right after dinner to start his homework and while he might start on time, he is easily sidetracked. For one thing, he keeps his computer on, and when his IM friends see he's on-line, they "drop by" for a chat. Eventually he'll get back to work, but then he might get a snack or hear the TV on and watch the Comedy Channel. He usually gets through most of his homework eventually, but the quality varies. His bedtime keeps getting later and later because he works so inefficiently, and his dad invariably yells at him about not getting to bed at a reasonable hour. Andy finds studying for tests is the worst. The night before a test he'll start studying, but after no more than 10 or 15 minutes, he'll decide he knows the material "as well as I'm ever going to" and will IM, play video games, or channel surf until he finds something to watch. His parents are very frustrated. They've considered depriving him of computer time or making him drop guitar, but they know both will trigger a huge fight. They dread that, and they're not sure it won't make things worse anyway.

After progress reports, his parents meet with his teachers and counselor, expressing their concerns. The parents and counselor discuss meeting with Andy to formulate a plan. At the meeting, his counselor tells Andy that she and his teachers feel he can do better, and he agrees. Reviewing what they see as distractions, the computer tops the list with TV probably second. The counselor reminds Andy and his parents that for middle school students the school recommends that computers be available when homework is complete. Andy uses his computer for some of his schoolwork. He proposes leaving an "away" message on his computer until 7:30 P.M. as a starting point, and his parents agree. Because he already sets aside time for homework, he agrees to set up a "schedule" so that he completes an assignment or part of an assignment before he takes a break. He thinks breaks of 10 minutes will work, and he will use a visible timer on his computer to keep track. To help him study for tests, he will meet with each of his teachers, and together they will develop a rubric outlining how to study in each subject along with estimated study time and a checklist to go with this. He also sets "reasonable" grade objectives for the next progress report so he, his teachers, and parents can evaluate his strategies. His parents will email his teachers weekly to check on late or missing assignments. Andy agrees to let parents "cue" him twice a night if he is off track, and they agree to use a cue phrase that he suggests.

Step 1: Establish Behavioral Goal

Target executive skill(s): Sustained attention

Specific behavioral objective: Andy will complete his assignments and study for tests to achieve his grade objectives for the quarter.

Step 2: Design Intervention

What environmental supports will be provided to help reach the target goal?
- Time-limited access to computer
- Visible time clock on computer
- Schedule for completion of assignments
- Rubrics from teachers for studying
- Two cues from parents
- Weekly feedback from teachers

What specific skill will be taught, who will teach the skill, and what procedure will be used to teach it?

Skill: Sustained attention to homework

Who will teach the skill? Parents and teachers

Procedure:
- Andy will use his computer for socializing and games after 7:30 P.M.
- Andy will set up an assignment schedule.
- He will allow himself timed 10-minute breaks.
- He will meet with teachers to establish study rubrics.
- Parents can cue him twice a night.
- Teachers will provide weekly performance feedback.

What incentives will be used to help motivate the child to use/practice the skill?
- Positive performance feedback from teachers

- Decreased conflicts with parents
- Improved grades

👍 Keys to Success 👍

- *Don't make any significant changes in the plan until your child has maintained improvements over one and preferably two marking terms (3 to 4 months).* It's not unusual for this plan to work initially, making parents and teachers overconfident that the problem has been solved permanently. But if you drop the plan altogether or become a lot less vigilant, your child's performance is likely to return, even if only gradually, to preplan levels. Then everyone involved usually concludes that the intervention didn't work.
- *Keep a reduced but still present level of monitoring in place for the whole year.* It may be hard to stick with it when things seem to be going so well, but it's only with this duration of reinforcement that many kids maintain long-term improvements in sustained attention.

Parent–Teacher Cooperation: Cutting Down on Distractions in School

Ellen never seems to get her second-grade work done. The problem began last year in first grade once students were expected to complete seatwork independently. Her teacher made some accommodations, such as reducing the workload, because Ellen was clearly a bright student who seemed to be able to master the lessons even though she couldn't always get her work done. This year's teacher is not so inclined, though, and work completion is becoming a bigger issue. Mrs. Barker, her teacher, first raised the issue at the parent–teacher conference that accompanied the end of the first marking period. "Ellen is such a social child," she said. "She seems to be able to keep track of everything else going on in the class and wants to help other students when they get stuck, but somehow can't find her way to getting through her own work."

Shortly afterward, Mrs. Barker started sending home with Ellen the work that she hadn't finished in school with the instructions to get it done for homework. Her mother finds herself spending long homework sessions with Ellen trying to get her through the work. This makes for a long day for both of them. Her mother feels that the daily homework assignments, which usually amount to about 10 minutes of math and 10 minutes of spelling, are reasonable, but when two or three unfinished worksheets are added on top of that, Ellen balks, and this often leads to frustration and tears. Ellen says she tries to get her work done in class, but she gets busy with other things. Her mother decides something needs to be done to address the fact that Ellen is not getting her work done in school.

Ellen and her mother meet with her teacher. They talk the problem over, and Mom says that at home Ellen seems to do better when she breaks jobs into smaller chunks and she sets a timer for Ellen. Her teacher says that 5 to 10 minutes is about the maximum amount of time that Ellen works before she gets distracted. She feels she can divide up Ellen's work into shorter blocks, but she's still concerned that Ellen will get distracted. They agree that when her teacher gives her independent work to do she will cue Ellen to set her timer. Her mother suggests that they make a checklist showing reading, math, and language arts work blocks. As soon as she finishes one part of the work she will give it to her teacher. Her teacher will praise her for the work completion, and Ellen can check off one block. Her teacher will give her the next part and cue her to set her timer. If she finishes before the other children and her teacher says her work is acceptable, she can engage in a preferred activity from a list she has made. Because socialization can be a distraction, during work time Ellen agrees she will move to a different area if cued by her teacher. If her work is not completed, she will use free time during the day or stay to complete it during homework club. Homework will continue to be completed at home. Mother and Ellen set up a system that gives her a sticker for each day her work is finished during class time. Ellen can then choose from a list of "special" activities once she earns a certain number of stickers.

Step 1: Establish Behavioral Goal

Target executive skill(s): Sustained attention

Specific behavioral objective: Ellen will complete assigned work in class within a specific time frame.

Step 2: Design Intervention

What environmental supports will be provided to help reach the target goal?

- Work will be divided into smaller blocks
- Timer and cues to set it
- Checklist for work
- Teacher cues

What specific skill will be taught, who will teach the skill, and what procedure will be used to teach it?

Skill: Sustained attention to work in class to increase work completion

Who will teach the skill? Teacher and mother

Procedure:

- Teacher agrees to break the work into smaller blocks of 5 minutes.
- Mother and Ellen buy a small timer for school.
- Teacher cues Ellen to set the timer at the beginning of work.
- Teacher and Ellen create a checklist for each subject work block.
- Ellen takes work to the teacher as soon as it's finished, the teacher praises her, and Ellen checks it off.
- Teacher gives Ellen the next work and cues her to set the timer.
- If Ellen finishes early, she can choose from a list of preferred activities.
- If socializing is a distraction, the teacher cues Ellen to move to a different area.
- Work not completed during class time will be done during free time or homework club.
- Ellen earns stickers at home for on-time work completion and can choose from a list of special activities when she earns a certain number of stickers.

What incentives will be used to help motivate the child to use/practice the skill?

- Praise from teacher
- Graph showing progress of on-time work completion
- Preferred activities in class for early work completion
- Stickers and special activities at home

👍 Keys to Success 👍

- *Make sure your child has the same assigned location in the classroom every day so the teacher knows that if she is not there, she's probably off-task.* We've used this system in public school classrooms for a number of years and found that success depends in good part on the teacher (or paraprofessional if there is one in class) maintaining the cueing and check-in system. The only way for this to be practical is for the student to be in a consistent location in the room.

- *Be sure to use an incentive system because it's the child who has to manage elements like setting the timer.*

- Make sure free time doesn't need to be used to complete work on a regular basis. This can be an effective strategy, but if it's needed all the time, you should meet with the teacher to determine where the plan has broken down.

15

....

Teaching Task Initiation

Task initiation is the ability to begin projects or activities without undue procrastination, in an efficient or timely manner. Adults have so many obligations that it might seem like all of us are good at initiating tasks—we have to be. Yet we know from our work with adults that this is not an easy skill for some people to develop, and even adults tend to put off until last the tasks they like least when a long to-do list is before them. This is not all that different from a child delaying homework until after playing one more video game—or leaving the least favorite homework assignment until the end of the evening. If procrastination and last-minute scrambling are particular problems for you, be sure to use the suggestions in Chapter 3 to increase your success when the two of you share this weakness.

How Task Initiation Develops

In the context of executive skills, task initiation does not apply to tasks we *want* to do but only to those we find unpleasant, aversive, or tedious—ones we have to *make ourselves* do. When children are preschool age, we don't expect them to start this kind of work on their own. Instead, we prompt them to do the task and then supervise them while they do it (or at least watch them get started).

Our first attempts as parents to get our children to begin tasks more independently comes through putting in place routines, such as morning or bedtime routines. Teaching your child that certain things have to be done at a set time each day in a set sequence is step one. Then, after a period of prompting and cueing (how long you need to do this will vary from child to child), your child internalizes the routine and is more likely to initiate it on his own or following a single reminder to "get started now."

Although it takes a long time to develop, task initiation is an important skill children need in school and beyond. Giving children developmentally appropriate chores to do is one of the best ways to begin teaching task initiation. Starting in preschool or kindergarten, this helps teach children that there are times when they have to set aside what they want to do in favor of something that needs to get done even though it may not be fun. This helps prepare them for school and for participation in extracurricular activities that sometimes necessitate setting aside preferred activities for something else.

In the questionnaire below, you can evaluate where your child might fall on the developmental ladder, based on the kinds of tasks children are capable of carrying out independently at various childhood stages. This scale helps you take a closer look at the assessment you did in Chapter 2, focusing on how well your child uses this skill.

HOW GOOD IS YOUR CHILD AT TASK INITIATION?

Use the following scale to rate how well your child performs each of the tasks listed. At each level, children can be expected to perform all the tasks listed fairly well to very well.

Scale

0—Never or rarely

1—Does but not well (about 25% of the time)

2—Does fairly well (about 75% of the time)

3—Does very well (always or almost always)

Preschool/kindergarten

_____ Will follow an adult directive right after it is given

_____ Will stop playing to follow an adult instruction when directed

_____ Can start getting ready for bed at set time with one reminder

Lower elementary (grades 1-3)

_____ Can remember and follow simple one- or two-step routines (such as brushing teeth and combing hair after breakfast)

_____ Can get right to work on a classroom assignment following teacher instruction to begin

_____ Can start homework at an agreed-upon time with a single prompt

(cont.)

Upper elementary (grades 4-5)

_____ Can follow a three- to four-step routine that has been practiced

_____ Can complete three to four classroom assignments in a row

_____ Can follow an established homework schedule (may need a reminder to get started)

Middle school (grades 6-8)

_____ Can make and follow a nightly homework schedule with minimal procrastination

_____ Can start chores at the agreed-on time (e.g., right after school)—may need a written reminder

_____ Can set aside a fun activity when he or she remembers a promised obligation

Teaching Task Initiation in Everyday Situations

• _Reinforce prompt task initiation throughout the day._ Prompt your child to begin each task she needs to do and praise her for starting right away or use an incentive system such as allotting points for beginning the task within 3 minutes of being asked, with the points redeemable for a desired reward. Of course you'll have to stay with your child long enough to make sure she gets started. You may also need to check back periodically to make sure she's still working on the task.

• _Provide a visual cue to remind your child to begin the task._ This could be a written reminder on the kitchen table so the child sees it when he gets home from school.

• _Break overwhelming tasks into smaller, more manageable pieces._ If the task seems too long or too hard, asking your child to do only one piece at a time may make her more likely to start on it.

• _Have your child make a plan for when or how the task will get done._ This gives him more ownership and control over the whole process and can have a dramatic effect on his ability to get started without excessive complaining or the need for multiple reminders.

• _Another way to give your child more ownership over the process is to have her decide how she wants to be cued to begin the task_ (for example, an alarm clock, a kitchen timer, or a naturally occurring event such as "right after dinner").

Doing It Now Instead of Later:
How to End Procrastination on Chores

Seven-year-old Jack is the middle of three children in his family. He has a 10-year-old sister and a 3-year-old brother. Both parents work full-time, and Jack's stepfather has to travel often for his job. With three children at home and Mom often the only caretaker, Jack's parents expect the children to help out around the house with tasks appropriate for their age. Because his brother is only 3, chores are primarily the responsibility of Jack and his sister. Once she understands what is expected, Emily doesn't need frequent prompts or reminders to get chores done. Jack is a different story. More often than not he requires frequent cues to begin the task. For example, it's his job to clear the dinner table and pick up toys in the living room before bed. At the very least, his mother has to nag him repeatedly, and sometimes he responds only when she gets angry and threatens loss of computer time. Once he does get started, as long as he understands what the task involves, Jack is pretty good about completing it. But getting him started is like pulling teeth. And at a recent school conference it became clear that Jack has the same difficulty at school, particularly with tasks that require a lot of effort, even though he's not struggling academically. His teacher has taken to giving Jack "start times" to begin work, which has helped him.

Jack's parents, knowing that work demands are only going to increase as he gets older, decide that now is the time to address the issue. Taking a cue from his teacher, his parents talk with Jack about having start times for two of his chores, clearing the table and toy pick-up. As an incentive they tell him that he can decide, within limits, how long before he starts a chore and he can pick out a time he likes from a few choices. Jack chooses a Time Timer, which uses a decreasing red clock face to show time remaining. They agree on a 5-minute delay for the table and a 10-minute delay for toys. Initially, parents will cue Jack by giving him the timer. He wants to manage keeping track of the elapsed time and beginning the task, and his parents agree. As a added incentive, for every 5 days that Jack begins his chore on time, he can have a "free pass," meaning he can skip one task for that day. If he doesn't start his chore within 2 minutes after the timer has gone off, he'll stop any other activity he is doing until the chore is complete.

At first, Jack's parents sometimes have to cue him to start once the timer goes off, but in general they see a definite improvement in his beginning tasks. After about a month, Jack no longer uses or needs the timer for clearing the table. They continue to use it for toy pick-up, although his parents notice that when Jack is told he has 15 minutes until bedtime, he often begins picking up at that point.

Step 1: Establish Behavioral Goal

Target executive skill(s): Task initiation

Specific behavioral objective: Jack will begin two chores after an agreed-on elapsed time with one cue.

Step 2: Design Intervention

What environmental supports will be provided to help reach the target goal?

- Jack will have a timer available to signal when to begin.
- Parents will provide a cue to set timer.

What specific skill will be taught, who will teach the skill, and what procedure will be used to teach it?

Skill: Task initiation on chores

Who will teach the skill? Parents

Procedure:

- Parents and Jack select the chores to practice the skill.
- Jack selects the start times for the chores.
- Jack chooses and parents buy a timer to signal the start time.
- Before each chore, his parents present the timer as a cue to set the time.
- Jack monitors the time, and when the timer signal occurs, he begins the task.
- If the chore is not started within two minutes of the timer signal, Jack stops any other activity until the chore is complete.

What incentives will be used to help motivate the child to use/practice the skill?

- Parent nagging is eliminated.
- Jack can earn a "free pass" for each 5 days of on-time task initiation.

👍 Keys to Success 👍

- *Be diligent about consistency during the initial "habit-building" period. When this intervention breaks down, it's usually because the system wasn't followed consistently in the first few weeks.*
- *Don't hesitate to reinstitute use of the cues and the timer for a few weeks if*

your child stops initiating assigned chores or other tasks over a period of a month or more. Sometimes kids need a refresher course.

- *If you find constant cueing or nagging necessary, impose loss of computer time or another valued privilege as a consequence.*

Laying the Groundwork for Success in High School and College: No More Procrastinating on Homework

It's about 4:30 on Tuesday afternoon and Colby, an eighth grader, has just arrived home after lacrosse practice. He lugs his heavy backpack into his bedroom and throws it down on his bed. He knows he should check his assignment sheets to remind himself what homework he has, but he spots his computer on his desk across the room and wonders if any of his friends are on-line. He tells himself he'll just check in, reminding himself he forgot to get the math assignment. Maybe it's on the homework website at school or one of his friends knows what it is. He turns on the computer, and IMs immediately begin to pop up. A friend asks if he's interested in a few rounds of an on-line game with a group that he sometimes plays with. He decides he'll play for a half hour and then get started on his homework. Around 5:30 his mother checks in with him to ask about his homework and to let him know they will eat at around 6:30. He assures his mother that he finished most of his work during his study period today and has only some social studies questions to complete. At 6:30 his father pops his head in to tell Colby that dinner is ready. Seeing that he's playing a video game, his father asks in an impatient tone when he's going to get to his homework. Colby, in a tone matching his father's irritability, says he has only a few social studies questions to answer and he'll take care of them after dinner. His father says nothing, not feeling like arguing tonight, but he's become more and more frustrated by the fact that Colby's grades don't match his ability. It seems to him that Colby always underestimates the amount of schoolwork that he has and the time needed to complete it and always overestimates the time he has available for other activities. To Dad, it's clear as day that Colby has memory and time management problems.

After dinner Colby finishes one of the social studies questions and is starting on the second when his friend calls. After half an hour, his father, exasperated, insists he get off the phone and finish his homework. Ten minutes later, he hangs up and returns to his homework. He alternates between social studies and IM and finishes the third question just before 9 P.M. Feeling good about the work he's done, he watches an episode of *South Park*, then reads a snowboarding magazine while in bed. Just before dropping off to sleep, he remembers the math assignment he didn't get to. He decides he can get to it tomorrow because he has lunch before math. His mother and father, having watched another night pass with their son spending time on nearly every activity but homework, wonder how his grades will look for this term.

A few weeks later, Colby receives the bad news in his progress report, with grades of B–, C, C–, and D in his main subjects. He and his parents meet with his counselor and eighth-grade team leader. Although Colby has statewide achievement test scores above the 90th percentile, his counselor reports that continued poor grades will exclude Colby from honors classes in high school. Colby has a few low quiz grades from surprise quizzes when he didn't read the material, but late and missing assignments account for the bulk of his poor performance. Colby resolves to do better, but his counselor, teacher, and parents are skeptical about the benefit of these good intentions, which haven't had a major impact in the past. Colby acknowledges this and agrees to consider other options.

His parents' past attempts to monitor his work were seen by Colby as (and typically were) "nagging," which led to bickering or fights. His counselor suggests that someone else might play this role, a kind of mentor or coach. Colby is willing to try this and identifies a teacher from last year he feels he could work with. His counselor has a plan for how coaching will work and, when approached by Colby, the teacher agrees to help. They meet for about 10 minutes at the end of each day to plan how Colby will manage his assigned work that night, and on at least 2 nights each week for the first 4 weeks the coach checks in with Colby by IM to see if he's following the plan. Colby and his coach also get weekly updates about late and missing assignments and his current performance from his teachers via email. By the end of the semester, Colby's grades have improved to B+, B, B, and C, and he and his coach decide to set a goal of all Bs or better for the next quarter.

Step 1: Establish Behavioral Goal

Target executive skill(s): Task initiation

Specific behavioral objective: Colby will complete his homework on time for 90% of assignments given without parental intervention or prompting.

Step 2: Design Intervention

What environmental supports will be provided to help reach the target goal?
- Colby will have a coach.
- Colby will meet with this person three times/week with additional phone contacts/emails as needed.
- Teachers will provide weekly feedback to Colby and his coach about late or missing assignments.

What specific skill will be taught, who will teach the skill, and what procedure will be used to teach it?

Skill: Task initiation on homework completion without parental reminders

Who will teach the skill? Coach

Procedure:

- Colby will choose a coach.
- Colby and the coach will establish grade objectives for next term.
- Colby, with help from the coach, will spell out any roadblocks to objectives.
- Colby and his coach will initially meet daily, and Colby will decide how much homework he has, how long it will take, and when he will do it.
- Colby and his coach will review the previous night's work as well as teachers' weekly feedback.
- Colby and the coach will talk by phone or IM at least three times a week to monitor his progress.

What incentives will be used to help motivate the child to use/practice the skill?

- Colby will improve his grades so that he is eligible for high school honors classes in at least two subjects.
- Colby and his parents will decrease daily arguments about homework by 75%.

👍 Keys to Success 👍

- *Be sure to find a coach who can work with your child and who is willing to make the brief but consistent daily contact (10 minutes and an IM message) and maintain this over a period of a least a few months.* At the middle school level we've seen teachers, counselors, paraprofessionals, and administrators all fill this role.

- *Institute a system of rewards and consequences if you have a dedicated coach but your child isn't following up on commitments made.* We've seen some kids actively avoid the coach or otherwise evade agreed-upon responsibilities, sometimes because their skill deficiency is severe and sometimes because no one is hovering over them when the time comes to do the work.

- *Make sure the coach gets feedback about how your child is doing with the plan.* When a coach doesn't know that a student's performance isn't improving or is

(cont.)

getting worse, he may not realize that he's not being consistent enough for a long enough time period to help the child gain the skill.

- *If you've tried the preceding tactics and your child is still not improving, you might consider another staff person as a coach.* Sometimes everyone is doing everything right, but the relationship between the student and coach just doesn't have that little something extra that motivates or teaches the child the necessary skill.

16

Promoting, Planning, and Prioritizing

The executive skill of planning/prioritization refers to the ability to create a roadmap to reach a goal or complete a task, as well as the ability to make decisions about what's important to focus on. We adults use this skill every day for brief tasks such as preparing a meal and for longer tasks such as launching a new project at work or arranging to have an addition put on the family home. If you can't identify priorities and then stick to them or create timelines for completing multistep projects, you may be the sort of person who tends to be seen as "living in the moment." Maybe you typically rely on others who are good at planning to help you achieve goals. If so, the suggestions in Chapter 3 will help you help your child despite having the same skill weakness.

How Planning and Prioritizing Skills Develop

When kids are very young, we naturally take on the planning role for them. We set up a task as a series of steps and prompt the child to perform each step—whether it's cleaning a bedroom or helping a child pack to go on a vacation or prepare for summer camp. Smart parents let children see this planning process on paper, creating lists or checklists for their kids to follow. Even when these lists are really for us, when our kids see us creating lists to organize work tasks, we're modeling desirable behavior that they will, if we're lucky, pick up for their own use. Written lists also reinforce what planning means by giving kids the opportunity to see what a specific plan actually looks like.

Planning becomes more critical in late childhood. It comes into play most prominently in school as children are given projects or long-term assignments with multiple steps, beginning around fourth or fifth grade. When teachers introduce such projects, they generally break down the assignment or project into subtasks and help students create timelines, often with deadlines attached. Teachers recognize that planning doesn't come naturally to children and, if left on their own, many will leave work until the last minute. Attaching interim deadlines forces students to complete larger projects in small chunks in a sequential fashion—the essence of planning.

By the time children hit middle school, they're often expected to perform this function more independently—and by high school this expectation extends beyond school assignments to the planning required to do things like find summer jobs and meet deadlines for SAT and college applications. Of course, some teenagers are better at this than others.

The second element included in this executive skill, prioritization, follows a similar pattern. Early in our children's lives we (and their teachers) decide what the priorities are and prompt kids to tackle the top priorities first. But beyond the high priorities that most adults would agree on—such as doing homework before settling down in front of the TV—how much leeway parents give their kids for prioritizing the use of their time often depends more on personal values than a desire to instill good prioritizing skills in their children. Our highly competitive world is full of kids whose every "free" moment is filled with dance or music lessons, sports, art classes, or religious studies because the parents—and sometimes the children—believe it's essential that their child be an accomplished achiever. We also see parents who believe—sometimes as a form of backlash to the prevalence of "overscheduled" kids—that "kids should be kids" and therefore don't encourage them to schedule their time at all. If left to their own devices too early in their lives, however, these children may end up frittering away their time watching television or playing video games. Naturally it's every family's right to promote the hopes and dreams they have for their children's achievements. But because the overall goal of enhancing your child's executive skills is to give the child what he needs to become independent, we've found it tends to work best when you take an active role in helping your child decide what the priorities are in the early years and gradually turn over that responsibility to the child as he gets older.

....

....
HOW WELL DEVELOPED ARE YOUR CHILD'S PLANNING SKILLS?
....

Use the following scale to rate how well your child performs each of the tasks listed. At each level, children can be expected to perform all the tasks listed fairly well to very well.

Scale

0—Never or rarely

1—Does but not well (about 25% of the time)

2—Does fairly well (about 75% of the time)

3—Does very well (always or almost always)

....

Preschool/kindergarten

_____ Can finish one task or activity before starting another

_____ Able to follow a brief routine or plan developed by someone else

_____ Can complete a simple art project with more than one step

....

Lower elementary (grades 1-3)

_____ Can carry out a two- or three-step project (e.g., arts and crafts, construction) of the child's own design

_____ Can figure out how to earn/save money for an inexpensive toy

_____ Can carry out a two- to three-step homework assignment with support (e.g., a book report)

....

Upper elementary (grades 4-5)

_____ Can make plans to do something special with a friend (e.g., go to the movies)

_____ Can figure out how to earn/save money for a more expensive purchase (e.g., a video game)

_____ Can carry out a long-term project for school, with most steps broken down by someone else (teacher or parent)

....

Middle school (grades 6-8)

_____ Can do research on the Internet either for school or to learn something of interest

_____ Can make plans for extracurricular activities or summer activities

_____ Can carry out a long-term project for school with some support from adults

....

Promoting Planning and Prioritizing
in Everyday Situations

- *Create plans for your child when young.* Use the expression "Let's make a plan" and then write it out as a series of steps. Better yet, make it a checklist, so the child can check off each step as it's completed.
- *Involve your child as much as possible in the planning process* once you've been providing models for a while. Ask, "What do you need to do first? And then what?" and so on and write down each step as the child dictates it to you.
- *Use things the child wants as a jumping-off point for teaching planning skills.* Children are likely more willing to make the effort to devise a plan to build a tree house than they might be to plan how to clean their closets, but the same principles apply in both cases.
- *Prompt prioritizing by asking your child what needs to get done first.* Ask questions like "What's the most important thing you have to do today?" You can also force this issue by withholding preferred activities until after the priorities are done (for example, "You can watch television when your homework is done" or "You can play video games once you've loaded the dishwasher").

Timelines and Deadlines:
Learning How to Plan Long-Term Projects

Max, age 13, is a good student who never had any problems with homework until the introduction of long-term projects when he was in fifth grade. At first he panicked, dreading the assignment from the day it was assigned until the day it was due. There were predictable emotional meltdowns whenever his mother brought it up and asked him what he'd done so far. As time went on, Max stopped telling his mother about the assignments at all, and she wouldn't know about it until his progress report came home or she got a note from the teacher informing her that Max had not handed in the assignment at all or what he'd done was hopelessly incomplete. His mother noticed he did better when teachers broke down the assignment into specific tasks and required students to complete and turn in each task on a specific due date. She also found that Max tended to do everything but the assignment, and when she asked about this, he always gave some reason that made sense to him: "I have to get my math done because Mr. Jones checks it off at the beginning of the period," or "I'm having a quiz on this short story in English tomorrow, so I have to finish reading it—you don't want me to fail the quiz, do you?"

Max's mother finally decided the stumbling block was that Max actually didn't know how to plan for a long-term project. She also felt that if any given component of the project was too complicated, that became a roadblock also. She got Max to agree to let her help him with the promise that if they planned right, the project wouldn't be so overwhelming to him. Using as a guide a timeline one of his teachers had put together for a project that Max finished without too much difficulty, she and Max identified the steps he needed to follow for a social studies project that was due in about 3 weeks. For each step they identified, she asked Max to estimate how difficult he thought that step was, using a scale of 1 to 10, with 1 being "a snap" and 10 being "just about impossible." They agreed that their goal was to make sure that each task felt like a 3 or less to Max. To make the whole thing a little more attractive, his mother also decided to build in incentives. Each time he completed a step on the day they had agreed on, he would earn 3 points. If he finished the step anytime before the agreed-upon deadline, he earned 5 points. Max had been wanting to get a new video game for quite a while, but it was expensive and he was having a hard time accumulating enough money to buy it when all he had to save was his allowance. Max and his mother agreed on how much each point was worth so that he could augment his savings and buy the video game sooner.

It took only one time through the process to be able to drop the incentive. Max's mother was pleased to see that each time they developed a plan, Max was able to do more and more of the planning himself.

Step 1: Establish Behavioral Goal

Target executive skill(s): Planning

Specific behavioral objective: To learn to plan and execute long-term school assignments

Step 2: Design Intervention

What environmental supports will be provided to help reach the target goal?

- Mother will assist in developing a plan and will supervise implementation (cueing, coaching).

What specific skill will be taught, who will teach the skill, and what procedure will be used to teach it?

Skill: To break down a long-term project into subtasks tied to a specific timeline

Who will teach the skill? Max's mother

Procedure:

- Make a list of steps required to complete the project.
- Assess how difficult each step is (using a 1–10 scale).

(cont.)

- Revise any step judged by Max to be more difficult than a 3 to make it easier.
- Decide on a deadline for each step.
- Prompt Max to complete each step.

What incentives will be used to help motivate the child to use/practice the skill?

- Points for completing each step on time (bonus points for completing it early)
- Points convert to money to help Max buy a video game he wants

👍 **Keys to Success** 👍

- *Don't hesitate to enlist the teacher's help if you feel you don't have the skill to start this intervention or the plan breaks down.* For this plan to succeed, you need the skill to help your child plan and to monitor the plan to make sure it's realistic and the agreed-upon timelines are followed. So here's a case where having the same weakness as your child can make success pretty elusive. You'll need the teacher's help in setting up work tasks and timelines. Sometimes teachers will feel that the project directions or rubric they've already provided already is sufficient. In that case, emphasize to the teacher that this is a weak skill area and that past performance indicates your child needs more specific and short-term tasks with regular monitoring and feedback.

A Social Director in the Making: Thinking Ahead about Getting Together with Friends

Alise is an active, social 7-year-old second grader. No kids her age live nearby, so if she's going to see friends outside of school, they have to come to her or she has to go to them. Her mom is happy to transport her if she is not tied up with work, driving her older siblings to drama or soccer, or other responsibilities. The trouble is that Alise doesn't think ahead far enough to make sure her friends are free and her mother is available before trying to arrange a play date. She'll get up on Saturday or Sunday morning and decide that she wants to have a friend over. But often her friends are busy or her mother has other obligations and can't drive Alise anywhere. Alise then ends up moping around the house in a bad mood, complaining that she has nothing to do. When she gets back to school on Monday, her friends will be talking about what they did with each other and she feels left out. Mom has repeatedly told her that she needs to make plans in advance. Alise agrees but typically does not remember to do it.

Mom suggests to Alise that they try to work out a solution, and she helps Alise through the planning process with a series of questions. "Suppose you wanted Jaime to come over. What's the first thing to do?" Alise responds, "I would ask Jaime in school if she wanted to come over." "Do you need permission to do that?" "Yes, I'll ask you first," Alise says. "Suppose she says yes. Then what happens?" "She comes over." "Does she need permission?" "Yes, I forgot that she has to ask her mother." "If it's okay with her mom, what do you need to decide next?" They continue on with this until they have a planning sequence, and with Mom's help Alise makes a list for herself.

Initially, her mom needs to cue Alise early in the week to think about a weekend plan, which means taking into consideration Mom's schedule as well as the activities her friends have. With practice, Alise is able to plan social events and even becomes something of a "social director" with her friends.

Step 1: Establish Behavioral Goal

Target executive skill(s): Planning

Specific behavioral objective: Alise will map out the steps to plan out-of-school activities with friends a few days in advance of the weekend.

Step 2: Design Intervention

What environmental supports will be provided to help reach the target goal?

- Parents provide questions/suggestions for activity-planning steps.
- List of steps to follow is completed.
- Mother cues Alise to start the planning process.

What specific skill will be taught, who will teach the skill, and what procedure will be used to teach it?

Skill: Planning for playdates

Who will teach skill? Mother

Procedure:

- Mom and Alise discuss steps to consider in planning a friend's visit.
- From this process, Mom helps Alise develop a written list of steps to follow.
- Mom cues Alise to begin the process before the weekend.

What incentives will be used to help motivate the child to use/practice the skill?

- Alise takes control of her social schedule and gets to have friends over.

👍 **Keys to Success** 👍

- *Figure out whether your child has reasonably good skills in task initiation and follow-through before undertaking a plan like this one.* If the plan fails as written, you'll need to provide significantly more prompting and direction to help your child get started. You could also check Chapters 14 and 15 to see if you want to try some of the ideas there for boosting your child's task initiation and sustained attention skills.

- *Make sure the problem with making play dates is not that your child is trying to make friends with a child who isn't a great match.* In our example, it's possible that some children are a better match for Alise than others. In that case, talking to the teacher could be really revealing. Ask the teacher which classmates she thinks are a good social fit for Alise and which may be less so.

- *Another option for boosting your child's social opportunities and enhancing planning at the same time is to look for regular, recurring activities on weekends.* Sports, drama, dance, and other programs can provide social opportunities in a scheduled, structured fashion that instills planning skills indirectly while ensuring that your child has predictable time with peers outside of school.

17

....

Fostering Organization

Organization refers to the ability to establish and maintain a system for arranging or keeping track of important items. For us adults the benefits of organizational abilities are pretty obvious. A system for keeping track of things and an orderly home or work environment eliminate the need to spend lots of time looking for things or neatening up just to get ready to work on something. We end up much more efficient as a result of having this skill. And this makes us less stressed. There's a reason why we tend to feel more comfortable when our surroundings have some degree of order and tidiness. Unfortunately, in our experience, adults for whom organization is a weak executive skill (and there are many!) find it quite challenging to improve their capacity. This makes it all the more critical that parents help their children develop organizational skills beginning at a fairly early age. We've provided some tips for teaching your child to be organized when you have a similar weakness in Chapter 3.

How Organizational Skills Develop

By now this pattern should sound familiar: At first, we provide our kids with organizational systems. We give them the structures they need to keep their bedrooms and playrooms neat, such as bookcases, toy boxes, and laundry hampers. We also supervise our children in maintaining tidiness. This means we neither clean our children's rooms for them nor expect them to clean their rooms on their own. Rather, parent and child work on room cleaning together, with the parent breaking the task down for the child ("OK, first we'll put all your dirty clothes in the laundry," "Now, let's put all your dolls on the doll shelf," etc.). We also establish rules such as "No eating food in the bedroom" and "Hang your coat up as soon as you come in from outdoors." But at first we don't expect kids to remember to follow the rules consistently—we assume they'll need reminders, and on those rare occasions when children remember to follow the rules without reminders we praise them lavishly.

Gradually we can step back from the step-by-step monitoring and supervision, getting by with a prompt in the beginning and a check at the end to make sure the child followed through. And somewhere around middle school or high school, children can take over maintaining organizational systems on their own. This doesn't mean that they won't need reminders from time to time—and the judicious use of withholding privileges can also be advantageous.

To assess how your child's organizational skills compares with his age group, complete the questionnaire below. This builds on the brief assessment in Chapter 2, helping you take a closer look at how well your child organizes things for his or her age.

HOW WELL DEVELOPED ARE YOUR CHILD'S ORGANIZATIONAL SKILLS?

Use the following scale to rate how well your child performs each of the tasks listed. At each level, children can be expected to perform all the tasks listed fairly well to very well.

Scale

0—Never or rarely

1—Does but not well (about 25% of the time)

2—Does fairly well (about 75% of the time)

3—Does very well (always or almost always)

Preschool/kindergarten

_____ Hangs up coat in appropriate place (may need a reminder)

_____ Puts toys in proper locations (with reminders)

_____ Clears place setting after eating (may need a reminder)

Lower elementary (grades 1-3)

_____ Puts coat, winter gear, sports equipment in proper locations (may need reminder)

_____ Has specific places in bedroom for belongings

_____ Doesn't lose permission slips or notices from school

Upper elementary (grades 4-5)

_____ Can put belongings in appropriate places in bedroom and other locations in house

_____ Brings in toys from outdoors after use or at end of day (may need reminder)

_____ Keeps track of homework materials and assignments

Middle school (grades 6-8)

_____ Can maintain notebooks as required for school

_____ Doesn't lose sports equipment/personal electronics

_____ Keeps study area at home reasonably tidy

Fostering Organization in Everyday Situations

There are two keys to helping children become better organized:

1. Put a system in place.
2. Supervise your child—probably on a daily basis—in using the system. Because this is labor intensive for adults—and because many children who have organizational problems have parents who are organizationally challenged—we generally recommend starting very small. Identify which domains are most important and work on them one at a time. As a practical matter, the highest priorities may involve schoolwork, such as keeping notebooks or backpacks organized or keeping a space clean for studying. Of lesser importance may be keeping closets or drawers clean.

Set up the organizational scheme carefully, involving your child as much as possible. If you and your daughter decide that keeping a desk clean is the priority, you may begin by taking her with you to an office products store and purchasing things like pencil holders, work baskets, or file cabinets and file folders. Once you and your daughter set up the desk as desired, make clearing off the desk part of the bedtime routine—initially, with on-site monitoring and supervision and eventually with reminders to start and check-ins when she's finished. You may find it helpful to take a photograph of the space when you first set it up, so your child has a model to compare her work to. The last step in the process might be for your daughter to look at the photo and see how closely her desk matches it.

We offer a note of caution for parents for whom organization is a particular strength. If you see your child as a "complete slob," you may need to modify your expectations—or at least your definition of "organized enough." We've found that many disorganized children are oblivious to the mess around them. They may never meet their parents' standard of neatness in part because they just don't see the disorder that is painfully apparent to Mom or Dad. Again, taking a photo of what's acceptable is a way to manage this—but before you take the picture, agree on the acceptable standard.

For a more detailed guide to help your child become organized, we recommend the book *The Organized Student* by Donna Goldberg.

Controlled Chaos: Getting Kids to Put Their Belongings Where They Belong

There were three children between the ages of 9 and 14 in the Rose family, and they all had an annoying habit of leaving their belongings wherever they were used last. They shed sweatshirts and sports equipment in the kitchen, toys tended to be strewn all over the living room, and they left dirty clothes in the bathroom after they showered at night. Mrs. Rose found that the clutter put her in a bad mood when she got home from a hectic workday and wanted to relax briefly before beginning dinner. She decided to call a family meeting to see if a solution could be found.

She began the meeting by describing the problem and the effect it had on her. The family then discussed how the kids might get in the habit of picking up after themselves and whether rewards or penalties might help. Mr. Rose suggested grounding whatever child left a mess, but everyone else felt that was too punitive. The kids suggested paying them for picking up after themselves, but that didn't feel right to their parents, and they weren't sure it would work anyway. They finally settled on a combination of rewards and penalties. The deal they worked out was this: At the beginning of every week, Mr. Rose put $25 worth of quarters in a jar. The kids agreed to pick up all their out-of-place belongings no later than 5:00 every afternoon when their mother got home from work. Any belonging out of place between then and bedtime would result in a quarter being removed from the jar. The belonging would be placed in a large plastic container in the laundry room, where it would remain off limits for 24 hours. If it was something that a child needed (like homework or a piece of sports equipment), the child could "buy" it back with some of his or her weekly allowance. At the end of the week, the family would count up the money remaining in the jar and decide how it would be spent.

Mrs. Rose left a small "white board" in the middle of the kitchen table with a reminder of the 5 o'clock deadline. On the white board she wrote the name of each child, and as they finished their work, they were to check off their names. Mrs. Rose also placed an alarm clock next to the reminder, and it was the job of the first child home from school to set the alarm for 4:30. When it went off, the kids stopped whatever they were doing and tidied up. Within a short time, they figured out they could divide up the work between them so it went more quickly. This approach also enabled them to hold each other accountable, so they could easily identify which child was not doing his or her share. They also started keeping an eye out during the evening for anything out of place and reminded each other to put things away.

Step 1: Establish Behavioral Goal

Target executive skill(s): Organization

Specific behavioral objective: To put away belongings in their appropriate places.

Step 2: Design Intervention

What environmental supports will be provided to help reach the target goal?

- Daily reminder and alarm clock on kitchen table when children get home from school

What specific skill will be taught, who will teach the skill, and what procedure will be used to teach it?

Skill: Organization

Who will teach the skill? Parents

Procedure:

- Set an alarm clock for 4:30 when the first child gets home from school.
- Cleanup process begins at 4:30 every day.
- Children work until the house is tidy, then check off their names on the white board.

What incentives/penalties will be used to help motivate the child to use/practice the skill?

- Monetary reward at the end of the week; loss of one quarter for each belonging out of place
- Loss of access to the belonging for 24 hours (opportunity to buy back the privilege using allowance)
- Group decision regarding how the money will be spent

👍 **Keys to Success** 🦴

- *If the system is too complex or breaks down, simplify it.* Especially if you're somewhat disorganized yourself, this system may be complicated to maintain for any length of time. In that case, set the time limit for pick-up as just before bed, making any item left out disappear for at least a day and any item redeemable for allowance. You also can base the money award individually so that each child who picks up gets money at the end of the day.

- *Make this a joint project if you're organizationally challenged too.* For example, agree that you'll clear off your kitchen counters or your own desk when your child is doing the same thing.

A United—and Organized—Front: Helping an Older Child Fulfill His Potential

Devon is a bright 14-year-old middle school student. For as long as he can remember, he has had difficulty organizing himself and routinely misplaces or loses things. Since entering middle school, the problem has gotten worse. He has more things to keep track of in and out of school, and his parents and teachers expect him to manage his belongings more independently. Therefore they're less willing than they were in the past to get him organized, search for his things, or replace them when he can't find them.

Until recently, his parents and teachers had adopted the approach of letting him suffer the consequences of his disorganization. If he lost his sports equipment, he couldn't play; if he lost his homework, he got a failing grade; if he lost some belonging, he had to earn the money to replace it. While they saw occasional improvements, these natural consequences did not resolve the problem. Devon's grades declined, his coaches got upset, and he lost some items he valued, such as his iPod. Devon became increasingly discouraged and felt more and more incompetent. His parents finally acknowledged that Devon clearly did not know how to solve the problem and it was time to offer some other kind of help.

Quickly they realized this was a major undertaking and was going to take additional work by Devon, his parents, and teachers. They decided to take on two areas: his homework because this was impacting grades and his room because he needed some consistent space to maintain any organization. For homework, they wanted a fairly simple system. His homeroom teacher agreed to check in with him in the morning to see if he had brought in his homework and in the afternoon to see if he had his assignments recorded and the materials he needed. His parents provided the teacher with a checklist that she would have Devon use and she would initial (see p. 245). Devon was typically conscientious about completing his homework, so all his parents needed to see was that Devon had put his homework in the homework folder and put the folder in his backpack.

Subject	HW handed in	Assignment written down	Materials in backpack
English			
Social Studies			
Science			
Math			
Spanish			

Room cleaning was more complicated. It had been Devon's decision to work on this, because he felt that if he could get his room organized and could keep it that way to some extent, he could better track his belongings. While he and his parents had worked on room cleaning from time to time in the past, they never made a systematic or long-term plan or made the same commitment to making it happen.

Devon and his parents agreed that rather than following their suggestions or schemes, it would be best if he came up with his own plan, getting assistance from them when he was stuck. He first took an inventory of his room and decided what categories each item fit into (shirts, pants, sports equipment, etc.). They then looked at what they had available for storage for different categories and what else Devon would need to organize everything and bought the various supplies. Although Devon agreed about the benefits of labeling these storage bins, he didn't want his friends to see the labels if they came over. So they compromised by making removable labels using Velcro.

Devon put in storage things that he didn't currently need but was unwilling to throw out, and his parents worked with him initially to help him get his room organized. They made up a checklist sequence he could follow to pick up his room and took pictures to serve as a model to compare the current state at any point with the ideal.

Devon realized that staying ahead of the clutter was critical. His parents initially agreed to remind him, but then he had the idea to place a cue on his computer that would remind him at least once a day to pick up. The real key to success, however, was a check-in by his parents every other day either after school or within an hour of waking on weekends to determine if he needed to pick anything up. If so, this would happen before he began to use his computer to IM friends.

As might be expected, over the course of months, while Devon did not maintain his original standard of organization, his room was significantly neater than prior to the system, and his parents were able to decrease cueing to once a week. The homework system also improved markedly, but everyone agreed that the afternoon teacher check-ins and the home check by the parents needed to continue.

Step 1: Establish Behavioral Goal

Target executive skill(s): Organization

Specific behavioral objectives: Devon will keep track of work handed out by his teacher, materials needed, and homework to be handed in. Devon will arrange his room according to categories of objects.

Step 2: Design Intervention

What environmental supports will be provided to help reach the target goal?

- Homework folders
- Checklist of assignments and materials
- Monitoring by parents and teacher
- Pictures of model room
- Storage bins with labels
- Cleaning sequence checklist
- Cueing by parents and computer

What specific skill will be taught, who will teach the skill, and what procedure will be used to teach it?

Skill: Organizing homework and room

Who will teach the skill? Teacher and parents

Procedure:

- Teacher checks for assignments recorded, materials needed, and assignments returned in folder.
- Parents check folder for presence of homework.
- Materials in room are categorized.
- Storage spaces are made available and labeled.
- Checklist for cleaning is developed and used.
- Parents monitor/cue and computer cues.

What incentives will be used to help motivate the child to use/practice the skill?

- Improved grades with on-time completion of work
- Retention of and ready access to belongings

👍 **Keys to Success** 👍

- *To increase the likelihood of success, begin with just one task.* We wrote the Devon story to show that different settings/tasks may be affected by weak organization and to demonstrate how strategies might be designed to address them. But realistically, addressing all of these at the same time would be labor intensive for your child, for you, and for your child's teacher(s). So consider picking one area—such as homework organization—getting that system up and running, and, after a month or two, moving on to another task.

18

....

Instilling Time Management

Time management is the capacity to estimate how much time one has, how to allo-cate it, and how to stay within time limits and deadlines. It also involves a sense that time is important. You probably know some adults who are great at time man-agement and some who aren't. Adults for whom this is a strength are on time for obligations, can estimate how long it takes to do something, and can pace their work depending on the time available (speeding up as needed). They tend not to overextend themselves, in part because they have a realistic sense of what they can accomplish. Adults who are weak at time management have difficulty sticking to a schedule, chronically "run late," and miscalculate when determining how long it takes to do anything. If you have these problems, see the suggestions in Chapter 3 for helping your child with a shared weakness.

How Time Management Develops

Because we know young children can't manage time, we do it for them. We prompt them to get ready for school or daycare, for example, allowing what we think will be enough time to complete the tasks at hand. Or we let them know what time they need to start getting ready for bed in order to have enough time to read a story after they've put on their pajamas, brushed their teeth, and washed up. If a special event is planned, we estimate how long it will take to get ready and cue children to do what they need to do so the family is ready on time. We notice that children work at different speeds, and we adjust our plans and prompts accordingly.

Gradually we give over the responsibility for this to our children. Once they've learned to tell time (somewhere around second grade), we can remind them to check the clock as they become more autonomous. When the day has predictable events built in, such as sports practice or favorite TV shows, we help children plan their time around those events. When we insist that children finish their homework or chores before going to a sports practice or before watching a television program, we're helping them learn to plan their time.

Sometimes kids hit a snag around middle school because the demands on their time increase just as we tend to cut back on monitoring and supervision. And the number of obligations increases right as the number of distracting activities also increases. How can you fit in homework when you want to play video games, IM, surf favorite websites, listen to newly discovered music, chat on cell phones with friends, and watch favorite TV shows? No wonder today's young people attempt to multitask! For some, the temptations are just too great, in which case we have to step back in and help them manage their time more effectively.

By high school, many young people have become more adept at juggling options and obligations and planning their time more effectively. If your children have not achieved this, it may be a cause for increasing friction between parents and teenagers because they are at an age where they resist direction and directives from parents.

HOW GOOD ARE YOUR CHILD'S TIME MANAGEMENT SKILLS?

Use the following scale to rate how well your child performs each of the tasks listed. At each level, children can be expected to perform all the tasks listed fairly well to very well.

Scale

0—Never or rarely

1—Does but not well (about 25% of the time)

2—Does fairly well (about 75% of the time)

3—Does very well (always or almost always)

Preschool/kindergarten

_____ Can complete daily routines without dawdling (with some cues/reminders)

_____ Can speed up and finish something more quickly when given a reason to do so

_____ Can finish a small chore within time limits (e.g., pick up toys before turning on the TV)

Lower elementary (grades 1-3)

_____ Can complete a short task within time limits set by an adult

_____ Can build in an appropriate amount of time to complete a chore before a deadline (may need assistance)

_____ Can complete a morning routine within time limits (may need practice)

(cont.)

....

Upper elementary (grades 4-5)

_____ Can complete daily routines within reasonable time limits without assistance

_____ Can adjust a homework schedule to allow for other activities (e.g., starting early if there's an evening Scout meeting)

_____ Can start long-term projects far enough in advance to reduce any time crunch (may need help with this)

....

Middle school (grades 6-8)

_____ Can usually finish homework before bedtime

_____ Can make good decisions about priorities when time is limited (e.g., coming home after school to finish a project rather than playing with friends)

_____ Can spread out a long-term project over several days

....

Instilling Time Management in Everyday Situations

• *Without going overboard, maintain a predictable daily routine in your family.* When children get up and go to bed at around the same time every day, and meals occur on a fairly set schedule, they grow up with a sense of time being an orderly progression from one event to another. This makes it easier for them to plan their time in between scheduled events (such as meals and bedtime).

• *Talk to your children about how long it takes to do things,* such as chores, picking up their rooms, or completing a homework assignment. This is the beginning of developing time estimation skills—a critical component of time management.

• *Plan an activity for a weekend or vacation day that involves several steps.* When you work with your child on planning skills, you're also working on time management because planning involves developing timelines for task completion. By talking with your child about "the plan for the day" and discussing how long it will take to complete the activity, your child is learning about time and the relationship between time and tasks. Doing this type of planning can actually be fun if you choose a fun activity, like spending the day with a friend. Ask the child to figure out how long it should take to have lunch, go to the park or beach, stop for ice cream on the way home, and so forth. The lessons learned will be especially meaningful to your child if he realizes that he and his friend got to pack the day with everything they wanted to do only because they blocked out their time in advance.

• *Use calendars and schedules yourself and encourage your child to do the same.* Some families post a large calendar in a central location where individual and family activities are posted. This has the effect of making time visible to your child.

- *Purchase a commercially available clock*, available from Time Timers (*www. timetimers.org*), that can be set to show visually how much time a child has left to work. Also described in Chapter 13, this device can be purchased in clock or wrist-watch form or as computer software.

Out of the House on Time: Managing Morning Routines

Seven-year-old Garret is the youngest in a family of four boys and has always desper-ately wanted to keep up with his older brothers. He wants to be independent, and when he was younger his favorite line was "I do it myself." Garret seems to under-stand the concept of time. He can tell time to the quarter hour and has a pretty fair idea of when his favorite shows are on TV. However, he often seems to lose track of time, and he has little sense of time urgency. This has led to problems at home and at school. At home, getting ready to go anywhere can be a major chore. Although the situation can be worse if the destination is a place that Garret doesn't want to go (for example, a doctor's appointment), he is slow getting ready even for preferred activities (for example, going to a water park). To get or keep him moving his par-ents or one of his siblings routinely cue or nag him. While this usually works eventu-ally, it's a source of growing frustration for family members. Garret doesn't struggle academically or exhibit any learning problems, but he's often the last to finish his work. His teacher has noticed that he can be more efficient when he needs to finish a task to get to a preferred activity such as recess.

His parents decide that Garret is old enough to begin to learn some basic skills in time management. They reason that if Garret is to learn how to finish tasks within a certain amount of time, he first needs to know what tasks are expected of him. Because leaving the house has been the issue, they decide to concentrate on the tasks he might need to complete to leave the house. This could range from the full-blown morning routine (wake up, get dressed, eat breakfast, brush teeth, etc.) to something as simple as getting his shoes on. Because the morning routine includes most of the "getting ready" tasks and he is slow in the morning, they decide to begin with this.

To take advantage of Garret's desire to be a "big boy" and be independent, they talk with him about a schedule of jobs in the morning. They try to sell the plan by telling him that if he can do his jobs on time, they won't have to nag him. Garret isn't particularly interested until they tell him he can earn prizes with this plan. He has fun making up the schedule, which consists of pictures and words, because he gets to "act" each scene (getting up, eating breakfast, brushing his teeth, etc.). His parents basically let him decide the order of the tasks on the schedule. They create a Velcro strip so that the order of the pictures can be changed and they can be removed. The plan is that as each job is finished, Garret will move that picture and put it in the "done" pocket attached to the bottom of the schedule. Rather than giving him a set time to begin with, over two mornings they agree that they will time him and use the result to decide how long he needs to finish. They make up a prize box with inexpensive little toys and treats (like gum) and put a picture of this at the end of the schedule. To increase his chances of success, his parents agree that for the first week or two they will check with him twice during the schedule as a reminder. His parents, after clearing it with the school, also insist that if he is slow in getting through his schedule and late for school as a result, he will make up the time either during recess or after school.

Using this system, Garret becomes more efficient and independent in the morning. For other "getting ready" times, his parents use a miniversion of this plan involving one or two pictures, the timer, and points that can be earned.

Step 1: Establish Behavioral Goal

Target executive skill(s): Time management

Specific behavioral objective: Garret will complete his morning routine tasks within a specific amount of time.

Step 2: Design Intervention

What environmental supports will be provided to help reach the target goal?

- Picture/written schedule with removable pictures
- Timer
- Cues from parents two times during the schedule
- Teacher support of the plan if he is late for school

What specific skill will be taught, who will teach the skill, and what procedure will be used to teach it?

Skill: Time management

Who will teach the skill? Parents/teacher

Procedure:

- Garret and his parents make up a visual/written schedule.
- Garret arranges activities in his preferred order.
- Parents set a timer in the morning.
- Parents check with Garret twice during his schedule.
- Garret removes a picture as each activity is completed.

- Garret chooses from the prize box if he gets through his schedule within the agreed-on time.
- If Garret is late for school, he makes up missed work during free time.

What incentives will be used to help motivate the child to use/practice the skill?

- Garret can choose an inexpensive treat from the prize box if he completes tasks on time.

👍 Keys to Success 👍

- *Keep a rough count of the number of cues you provide and how close you need to be (in the doorway vs. at the bottom of the stairs, for example) to make your reminders effective.* Twice during the schedule may prove not to be enough. You may need to issue more reminders to get your child used to getting the assigned tasks done during the allotted time. Although it can be somewhat annoying to keep this kind of record, it will allow you to see progress and appreciate the pace needed to wean your child from these supports. Without having this sense of progress, parents often feel the system isn't working and go back to nagging.

Time Warp: Learning to Estimate How Long a Task Will Take

Nathan's parents have always appreciated the eighth grader's mellow nature, which contrasts so sharply with his sister, who panics every time she has a test to study for. But ever since he entered middle school, his parents have become increasingly concerned about his tendency to put off homework until too close to bedtime, which means he rushes through it or may not finish it all. Problems are compounded when he has long-term projects because he often leaves them until the day before they are due. Over time, his mother has realized that part of the problem is that Nathan has no idea how long things take to do. A paper he thinks he can write in half an hour may take him 2 hours, and a project he thinks he can put together in a couple of hours may take 5 or 6. His parents have tried repeatedly to get Nathan to understand that his ability to estimate time is weak, but even when he acknowledges the fact that the last time he wrote a paper it took him 2 hours, this time, because he knows what he wants to write about and has a rough outline in his head, he's sure he can whip it out in an hour max.

After one too many arguments when his parents pointed out yet again that he was no judge of time and Nathan told them in no uncertain terms to "Get off my case!" his parents decided they had to figure out another way to handle the problem.

They took Nathan out to dinner on a Saturday night when he wasn't doing any-thing with friends and proposed that each day when he got home from school he make a list of the homework assignments he had to do that night and estimate how long each assignment would take. He would then decide at what time he was going to start his homework based on his estimates, with the understanding that he would be done by no later than 9:00. If he was off by more than 20 minutes, then the next day he would start his homework at 4:30. If his estimates were accurate, then he could determine what time he would start his homework the next day. They also agreed he had to build in time to study for tests and to do a little work on long-term projects at least two to three nights a week unless his daily homework took more than 2 hours. Nathan agreed to this plan because he thought it would give him a chance to prove his parents wrong—he even spent an hour on the computer when he got home, happily creating a spreadsheet he could use to keep his data. He told his mom he would email the spreadsheet to her as soon as he filled out his daily plan. They agreed that she would check the plan and would check in with him at the time he said he would be done with his homework, at which point he would show her all the assignments he had completed.

For the first couple of weeks his mom needed to remind Nathan to make the plan and email it to her. Nathan quickly learned that he wasn't as good at estimat-ing as he thought he was. But because he hated starting his homework so soon after he got home from school, he gradually improved his ability to estimate how long homework would take. A couple of times, when he showed his parents his work, they saw that he'd done a rather sloppy job, apparently in an effort to get it done on time. They talked about introducing a penalty for sloppiness, and with a warning that this would happen if sloppiness became an issue, Nathan cleaned up his act—at least enough so his parents decided not to push the issue.

Step 1: Establish Behavioral Goal

Target executive skill(s): Time management

Specific behavioral objective: Nathan will learn to accurately estimate the time needed to complete homework by a specific time each night.

Step 2: Design Intervention

What environmental supports will be provided to help reach the target goal?

- Start and stop times for homework
- Spreadsheet for estimated work times
- Check-ins with mother

What specific skill will be taught, who will teach the skill, and what procedure will be used to teach it?

Skill: Time management

Who will teach the skill? Parents/Nathan

Procedure:

- Nathan will make a list of homework assignments and the estimated time needed to complete them, put this on a spreadsheet, and send it to his mother.
- Based on these estimates, he will decide what time to begin homework.
- Work will be completed by 9:00 P.M., and if his estimate is off by 20+ minutes, he will start work earlier the next day.
- Nathan will build in time to study for tests and will commit to work on long-term projects two to three nights per week.

What incentives will be used to help motivate the child to use/practice the skill?

- Nathan can manage his own time without interference or nagging from parents.

👍 Keys to Success 👍

- *Vigilance from you is critical in the early stages of the intervention because most kids will find some elements of the plan require a lot of effort and will therefore forget or avoid them.*
- *Have the child's teachers independently verify the amount and quality of work completed by the child.* As designed, this plan requires accurate reports from the child. In our experience, the most effective way to prevent breakdown of the plan is to have the teachers offer feedback, probably by email. Reports should come to you, with a copy to your child.

19

Encouraging Flexibility

The executive skill of *flexibility* refers to the ability to revise plans in the face of obstacles, setbacks, new information, or mistakes. It relates to an adaptability to changing conditions. Adults who are flexible are able to "go with the flow." When plans have to change at the last minute due to variables beyond their control, they quickly adjust, to problem solve the new situation and to make the emotional adjustment necessary (such as overcoming feelings of disappointment or frustration). Adults who are inflexible are often described as being "thrown for a loop" when circumstances change unexpectedly. Those who live with inflexible individuals, whether adults or children, often find it takes extra energy and planning on their part to reduce the impact of unexpected change on the inflexible family member. If you're no more flexible (or only a little bit more) than your child, you'll find suggestions in Chapter 3 that will help you compensate for the shared weakness so you can help your child optimally.

How Flexibility Develops

We don't expect babies to be flexible about anything. So we accommodate their schedules, feeding them when they're hungry and letting them sleep when they're tired. Fairly early on, however, parents begin to introduce more order and predictability so that they no longer have to ignore the schedules of the outside world to satisfy their baby's needs. By 6 months of age, for instance, most infants are following the sleep schedule of the family (that is, sleeping through the night as much as possible). Eventually, especially as solid food is introduced, we shape mealtimes as well so they align more closely with family mealtimes.

As children progress from infancy to toddlerhood to the preschool years, we expect them to be flexible in a variety of situations—and most are. These include adjusting to new babysitters, starting preschool, and spending the night at a grand-parent's house. We also expect them to adjust to unexpected changes in routines, deal with disappointments, and manage frustrations with a minimum of fuss. All these situations require flexibility, and some children handle them better than others. For the majority of children who struggle, parents find that it takes them a while to adjust to new situations, but they eventually do, and the next time a similar situation arises, it takes them a little less time to adjust. Somewhere between the ages of 3 and 5, most children have learned to manage new situations and unexpected events and either take them in stride or recover quickly if upset.

HOW FLEXIBLE IS YOUR CHILD?

Use the following scale to rate how well your child performs each of the tasks listed. At each level, children can be expected to perform all the tasks listed fairly well to very well.

Scale

0—Never or rarely

1—Does but not well (about 25% of the time)

2—Does fairly well (about 75% of the time)

3—Does very well (always or almost always)

Preschool/kindergarten

_____ Can adjust to a change in plans or routines (may need warning)

_____ Recovers quickly from minor disappointments

_____ Is willing to share toys with others

Lower elementary (grades 1-3)

_____ Plays well with others (doesn't need to be in charge, can share, etc.)

_____ Tolerates redirection by teacher when not following instructions

_____ Adjusts easily to unplanned situations (e.g., a substitute teacher)

Upper elementary (grades 4-5)

_____ Doesn't "get stuck" on things (e.g., disappointments, slights, etc.)

_____ Can "shift gears" when plans have to change due to unforeseen circumstances

_____ Can do "open-ended" homework assignments (may need assistance)

(cont.)

Middle school (grades 6-8)

_____ Can adjust to different teachers, classroom rules, and routines

_____ Is willing to adjust in a group situation when a peer is behaving inflexibly

_____ Is willing to adjust to or accept a younger sibling's agenda (e.g., allowing him/her to select a family movie)

Encouraging Flexibility in Everyday Situations

Especially when you're first working on this skill, you'll need to emphasize environmental modifications if your child has significant problems with flexibility. Youngsters who are inflexible have difficulty handling new situations, transitions from one situation to another, and unexpected changes in plans or schedules. Therefore helpful environmental modifications include:

- Reducing the novelty of the situation by not introducing a lot of change all at once
- Keeping to schedules and routines whenever possible
- Providing advance warning for what's coming next
- Giving the child a script for handling the situation—rehearsing the situation in advance and walking the child through what's likely to happen and how she can use her script
- Reducing the complexity of the task. Inflexible children often panic when they think they won't remember everything they have to or when they think they won't succeed at what they're expected to do. Breaking tasks down so that they have to do only one step at a time will reduce the panic.
- Giving children choices. For some children, inflexibility arises when they feel someone is trying to control them. Offering choices for how to handle situations returns some of the control to them. Obviously, you'll have to be able to live with whatever choice the child makes, so you need to consider carefully the options you present.

As your inflexible child matures, you can use the following strategies to encourage greater flexibility:

- _Walk your child through the anxiety-producing situation,_ offering maximum support initially so he never feels he is "on his own" in tackling the task. As he achieves success, confidence grows naturally, and the support is faded gradually. This approach is actually one that parents use all the time to help children adjust to new or anxiety-provoking situations. If your child has never gone to a birthday party and is apprehensive about it, you don't just drop him off and pick him up 2 hours later. You go in with him and stay for a while, until he's comfortable, and then you gradually pull yourself back and eventually leave the party. If your child is afraid of going into the water at the beach, you go in with her at first, holding her hand and letting her know you won't let go until she's ready. In other words, you provide physical support or your presence initially and then melt into the background as your child develops a comfort level and the confidence that he or she can manage the situation alone. The key is (and this should sound familiar) *offering the minimum support necessary for the child to feel successful.*

• *Use social stories to address situations where the child is predictably inflexible.* Social stories, developed by Carol Gray as a way to help children with autism understand social information so they can handle social interactions more successfully, can be used to help children with executive skill weaknesses as well. Social stories are brief vignettes that include three kinds of sentences: (1) descriptive sentences that relate the key elements of the social situation; (2) perspective sentences that describe the reactions and feelings of others in the situation; and (3) directive sentences that identify strategies the child can use to negotiate the situation successfully. For more information about social stories, visit Carol Gray's website (*www.thegraycenter.org*).

• *Help your child come up with a default strategy for handling situations where her inflexibility causes the most problems.* These include simple measures like counting to 10, walking away from the situation to cool off and then returning, and asking a specific person to intervene.

• *Use some of the coping strategies* in *What to Do When Your Brain Gets Stuck*, by Dawn Huebner. Although the book is written for children with an extreme form of inflexibility, obsessive–compulsive disorder, it offers some nice descriptions of what it feels like to be inflexible as well as good coping strategies. As with the other books by Dawn Huebner mentioned earlier, this book is meant to be read by parents and children together and is intended for children ages 6–12.

The Lone Ranger: When a Teen Tries to Take Control of All of Her Own Plans

Anna is a 14-year-old eighth grader. She has always done better when she knows well in advance what is expected of her and what events or activities are scheduled. It's not unusual for her to have a meltdown when faced with unexpected changes in plans. Because Anna is older now, she has more opportunity to make her own plans and decisions, which she likes. Her parents see the upside and downside to this. The upside is that there are somewhat fewer conflicts because they are directly involved in fewer decisions. The downside is that Anna often makes decisions and plans without checking with her parents, even though the plans require parental involvement or consent. For example, in the most recent 2 months, she has invited friends for a sleepover, made plans to go to a party, and agreed to hang out with a friend at a video arcade. In each case she did not check with her parents, and she exploded when told either that her plan could not happen or that they needed more details before giving permission. Anna's parents also get this reaction if they forget to give her advance warning (usually a day or two) about things like doctor or dentist appointments. As she has entered adolescence, the explosions have become more intense, with Anna screaming, throwing things, and telling her parents that she "hates" them. Depending on her behavior, her parents may end up grounding her, but this has not resolved the problem. The issue seems to involve Anna setting a plan or agenda for how she will spend her time without realizing or considering that other people may have different plans. Once she sets her plan, anyone else's plan is an unexpected change, and she reacts negatively as she always has.

In a calm moment, Anna and her parents talk and agree that they don't like the way things are going now. Anna says she would like more freedom in making choices. Her parents would like Anna to consider their plans and schedules as well as some basic rules they expect her to follow when she makes plans. Knowing that Anna does best with predictable routines and expectations, they propose the following:

- On days after school when she does not have a scheduled activity (such as play practice or an appointment) she can choose one of her "regular" activities— library, friend's house, or school game. She needs to call her mother to say where she is going, with whom, and how she will get there. When she arrives at the place, she will call her mother to let her know. If it's a friend's house, Mom will speak with the friend's parent. Once at a place, she cannot leave without permission, and her mother will pick her up or she will tell her mother who is going to drive her home. If she does not abide by these rules, she will forfeit her privilege (that is, the chance to do one of her regular activities) for a week.

- For special activities like dances, trips to mall, sleepovers, and parties, Anna cannot participate unless she gets permission, which won't even be considered unless Anna tells them where she is going, with whom, for how long, and what the transportation is. She also needs to say who will supervise, and parents will talk to this person to check.

- Because communication is a key element of this plan, her parents agree to get Anna a cell phone, and she agrees not to use it during school hours.

- For appointments or activities they schedule for Anna, her parents will let her know at the time that they schedule these and also remind her 2 days before the appointment.

- At least twice a week Anna and her parents will review the plan and decide whether any changes need to be made.

Along with this plan Anna's parents explain why having this information is important to them. She feels that they are more careful than they need to be, but she's willing to give the plan a try.

Step 1: Establish Behavioral Goal

Target executive skill(s): Flexibility

Specific behavioral objective: Anna will inform her parents if she chooses an agreed-on activity or will ask permission before committing to activities that have not yet been agreed upon.

Step 2: Design Intervention

What environmental supports will be provided to help reach the target goal?

- Anna will have a list of "preapproved" activities.
- Her parents will provide Anna with a cell phone.
- Her parents will give Anna advance notice of appointments.

What specific skill will be taught, who will teach the skill, and what procedure will be used to teach it?

Skill: Anna will learn to take other people's agendas into consideration when making her own plans and will accept limits on her own plans.

Who will teach the skill? Parents

Procedure:

- Anna can choose from a list of activities that do not require advance permission and will let her parents know her choice.
- Activities outside this list always require that Anna get advance permission.
- Anna will communicate with her parents using a cell phone they provide.
- Her parents will give Anna advance notice of appointments/obligations they schedule for her.
- Anna and her parents will meet twice a week to evaluate the plan.

What incentives will be used to help motivate the child to use/practice the skill?

- Anna will have increased control/choice over some activities.
- Anna will have advance notice of appointments.
- Anna will get a cell phone.

👍 **Keys to Success** 👍

- *Do your best to stick to the original agreement and follow through with consequences.* It would not be unusual for a 14-year-old to test/push the limits of this plan by not calling, calling late, or making a tentative plan and then running it by her parents. This could be accidental (forgetting to call) or intentional. It can be difficult to hold the line when this happens because it's natural to want to give your child more chances or to want to avoid a major tantrum. But unless you're consistent, this intervention won't get you and your child anywhere.

Handling Changes in Routines

Manuel is 5. He attends the afternoon kindergarten session, and his mother picks him up at 2:30 each day. Manuel has always been a creature of habit. His parents, who are not naturally organized, have learned that regular routines and organized spaces are important for Manuel. Getting him to try new activities requires a lot of coaxing, and he won't give something new a second chance if his first experience ends up at all negative. When he started to tip over while riding a bike without training wheels, he refused to try riding again even though his dad caught him. In school it took a while, but he plays with peers and seems to enjoy himself. However, in other social situations with peers or adults, unless they're very familiar, Manuel tends to hide behind his mother or father. The afternoon pick-up schedule can sometimes be a major problem for Manuel and his mother. They've established a regular routine for most days. After Mom picks him up, they stop for a snack at a nearby store. She puts a CD in that he likes to listen to, and they ride home the long way so he can finish his snack. If the weather is good, he plays in the yard, and if not he builds with blocks in the basement. Any change in this afternoon—stopping at the bank, picking up his sister at school, or taking her to an activity—makes Manuel cry and throw things, and he stays upset for a few hours. Although Manuel's mother understands his need for routine, she's tired of these outbursts. She understands that as he grows older, neither the family nor the rest of the world will be able to accommodate his routines and they need to come up with strategies to increase his tolerance for change.

The issue seems to be that Manuel is fixed on one plan or outcome when he's picked up. His mother decides to try getting him used to a few different pick-up plans on a regular basis. She knows that surprises don't work for him, so first she introduces the idea: "Manuel, sometimes after I pick you up we get your snack and come home. Sometimes I have to do something before we come home, like stop at the bank or pick up Maria. Most of the time, I know the night before. How would you like me to let you know? I can just tell you or we could make up a plan using pictures." Manuel would rather nothing change, but his mom is determined, and he chooses pictures. They decide that they may eventually take photos. But to start, with his sister's help, he draws pictures of the car, home, the bank, Maria's school, and Maria playing soccer because these are the most likely stops. They put clear contact paper over each picture and Velcro the backs. Manuel's mother starts with changing the routine two days each week and then moves to three. Each night she and Manuel talk about what the plan for the next day is and he arranges the pictures into a "schedule." Before he goes to school the next day, they go over the schedule and she takes it with her in the car for the end of school. At first Manuel protests when it's a different day, but the protests are mild in comparison to before. Over time, Mom adds other errands and Manuel seems to have less and less difficulty with these after-school changes as long as he gets some advance warning. Mom is able to move the warning time to the morning, before he leaves for school that day. Her goal eventually is to give Manuel the plan or schedule when she picks him up because this would allow her to be flexible in planning her day.

Step 1: Establish Behavioral Goal

Target executive skill(s): Flexibility

Specific behavioral objective: Manuel will participate in schedule changes for his after-school pick-up without tantrums.

Step 2: Design Intervention

What environmental supports will be provided to help reach the target goal?

- Manuel has pictures of possible after-school activities.
- Mother tells Manuel about the plan the night before.
- Mother reviews the schedule in the morning and takes it with her for pick-up.

What specific skill will be taught, who will teach the skill, and what procedure will be used to teach it?

Skill: Flexibility around schedule changes

Who will teach the skill? Mother

Procedure:

- Mother tells Manuel that there will be schedule changes and asks him how he would like to be informed about these.
- Pictures of different activities are made.
- For each day, depending on the plan, the pictures are arranged into a schedule.

(cont.)

- The schedule is reviewed the night before, the day of, and in the afternoon when Manuel gets in the car.
- New activities/changes are added over time.

What incentives will be used to help motivate the child to use/practice the skill?

- No specific incentives are included in the plan.

👍 Keys to Success 👍

- *Don't expect your child to be flexible about changes in the intervention!* Remember, you're dealing with a child who has great difficulty with changes in daily routines. Once this new system is in place, it too can become a fixed expectation for the child. This means that if you don't use it, you might have to deal with a tantrum about changes in the intervention itself. Any significant change in the plan should be reviewed with the child so he knows what's coming.

- *Be prepared to add unheralded changes to the intervention.* Sometimes you just can't anticipate a change far enough ahead to prepare your child, yet she needs to learn to roll with these changes too. Once your child is demonstrating some ability to handle changes in schedule with equanimity, tell her well beforehand that on-the-spot changes can happen once in a while. Then start introducing some last-minute changes in the schedule, but stick to ones your child will like, such as going to get ice cream, at first. Then gradually introduce other types of changes.

20

....

Increasing Goal-Directed Persistence

Goal-directed persistence refers to setting a goal and working toward it without being sidetracked by competing interests. Anytime we keep striving to reach a long-term goal we're exhibiting this skill. A 25-year-old who decides she wants to run a marathon and trains for a year to do that shows good goal-directed persistence. A store clerk who decides he wants to become a manager and volunteers for additional jobs at work to show he has the motivation to work his way up also has goal-directed persistence. And when couples cut back on recreational and entertainment expenses to save up enough money for a down payment on a house, they, too, are showing goal-directed persistence. If you find yourself changing your goals a lot in response to new interests that arise or you don't consider improving your performance over time important, you may suffer from a skill deficit in goal-directed persistence and can use the suggestions in Chapter 3 for making the most of your efforts to help your child when you share your child's weakness.

How Goal-Directed Persistence Develops

Although goal-directed persistence is one of the last executive skills to mature, from the time your child was quite young you've been encouraging the development of this skill—even if you've never recognized it as such. Whether it's helping your toddler put together a puzzle or helping your 5-year-old learn to ride a bike, every time you've encouraged your child to keep trying even when something is hard you've given her goal-directed persistence a nudge forward. Likewise, when you impress upon your child that mastering new skills takes time, practice, and effort, and you praise your child for sticking with something tough, you've helped the child value goal-directed persistence. Most notably, children learn the idea of persistence through sports or learning a musical instrument, but you also teach persistence by assigning tasks such as chores. In the beginning, chores are kept brief and contained within a small space (like putting away one's toothbrush or hanging up one's coat). As your child has gotten older, you've naturally recognized that he could handle longer chores or those that demand working in larger spaces (cleaning his room, raking leaves, walking the dog, and the like).

Giving your child an allowance and helping him learn to save money for desired objects is another way you help your child develop goal-directed persistence. By third grade, most children have learned to save at least a little money toward something they want to buy. By the time they reach middle school, a majority of children have learned the concept of goal-directed persistence at least well enough to practice a sport or a musical instrument or to make choices about how they spend their time in order to earn good grades in school. By early high school, youngsters are beginning to understand that their daily performance in school can affect outcomes such as college choices, and by late sophomore year or the beginning of their junior year, they may be taking bigger steps to alter their behavior to achieve desired long-term goals.

To assess how your child's goal-directed persistence compares with her age group, complete the questionnaire below, which builds on the simpler assessment you did in Chapter 2.

HOW GOOD IS YOUR CHILD AT GOAL-DIRECTED PERSISTENCE?

Use the following scale to rate how well your child performs each of the tasks listed. At each level, children can be expected to perform all the tasks listed fairly well to very well.

Scale

0—Never or rarely

1—Does but not well (about 25% of the time)

2—Does fairly well (about 75% of the time)

3—Does very well (always or almost always)

Preschool/kindergarten

_____ Will direct other children in play or pretend play activities

_____ Will seek assistance in conflict resolution for a desired item

_____ Will try more than one solution to get to a simple goal

Lower elementary (grades 1-3)

_____ Will stick with a challenging task to achieve the desired goal, such as building a difficult Lego construct

_____ Will come back to a task later if interrupted

_____ Will work on a desired project for several hours or over several days

Upper elementary (grades 4-5)

_____ Can save up allowance for 3-4 weeks to make a desired purchase

_____ Can follow a practice schedule to get better at a desired skill (sport, instrument)—may need reminders

_____ Can maintain a hobby over several months

Middle school (grades 6-8)

_____ Able to increase effort to improve performance (e.g., work harder to get a higher grade on a test or a report card)

_____ Willing to engage in effortful tasks in order to earn money

_____ Willing to practice without reminders to improve a skill

From _Smart but Scattered_ by Peg Dawson and Richard Guare. Copyright 2009 by The Guilford Press.

Increasing Goal-Directed Persistence in Everyday Situations

While this skill is one of the last executive skills to develop fully, there are steps you can take beginning when your child is quite young to help him develop goal-directed persistence:

• _Start very early, beginning with very brief tasks where the goal is within sight_ (in terms of time and space). Offer assistance to help the child complete the task and praise her for getting the task done. For instance, one of the earliest games children enjoy are puzzles. Begin with puzzles with very few pieces, and if the child gets stuck, give her cues or assistance (for example, point to the piece the child needs and the place it needs to go and have the child put the piece in place).

• _As you help your child stretch and reach more distant goals, begin with ones that the child wants to work on._ Your son will likely be more interested in persisting with a task such as building a more complicated Lego structure than he is in cleaning up his bedroom floor. Encourage him, provide small cues, hints, and assistance as needed (the minimal help necessary for the child to be successful), and then praise him for sticking with it.

• *Give your child something to look forward to doing when the chore is finished.* This will encourage your child to persist with tasks that aren't so much fun, such as chores. If your child's stamina is pretty low, provide a reward after part of the chore is completed.

• *Gradually build up the time needed to reach goals.* At first the goals should be reachable within a few minutes or in less than an hour. The amount of time can be increased, and eventually your child will be able to go longer before achieving the goal or earning the reward. To help her learn to delay gratification for minutes to days, build in concrete feedback about her progress toward the goal. Tokens in a jar, puzzle pieces, coloring in sections of a drawing—all of these can be used to represent progress (not unlike the thermometers often used for community fundraisers, where the amount of money raised is reflected by the mercury in the thermometer).

• *Remind the child what he is working toward.* If he's saving money for a toy, place a picture of the toy on his bedroom wall or the refrigerator door. Visual reminders are generally more effective than verbal reminders. Verbal reminders are often interpreted as nagging by thin-skinned adolescents!

• *Use technology to provide the reminders.* One example is the Post-it notes that appear on the desktop when the computer screen is turned on; there are also "countdown" programs such as the one available as a widget download for Macintosh computers.

• *Make sure a reward you use as incentive for goal-directed persistence is one your child really wants and doesn't have free access to.* If you have a child who loves video games, for instance, and who has three different game systems, two dozen games, and can play them whenever she wants, she's not going to be too motivated to delay gratification and persist toward any goal to get video games or game time.

Quitters Never Win Self-Confidence: How to Help a Child Stick with Work and Play

Five-year-old Samuel is a curious kindergartner who likes to try new things, but he seems quick to abandon every activity, either from loss of interest or because it's too hard. He gives up on "work" tasks such as simple chores and school activities but also on the fun stuff, like video games and athletics (hitting/catching a ball, riding a bike). Samuel's 3-year-old sister is a "bulldog" who will persist until she achieves whatever she set out for, which makes Samuel's parents worry even more about their son. Will his lack of persistence make him more passive and less open to new activities? He already seems less confident than he was when younger.

Samuel's parents want to help him, but neither encouragement during an activity nor insistence that he finish has had a lasting impact. They would like to make a plan with Samuel, but they need some additional information. When Samuel starts an activity, are his expectations too high? Once he starts, does his goal seem too far off? After talking with Samuel about some activities that he has put aside, they realize both factors can come into play. With baseball he wanted to hit a "home run" (off the tee and out of the yard) when he batted. After a few failures he thought he'd never get there, so he stopped.

Samuel's dad offers to help him with hitting if Samuel agrees on shorter, easier goals (such as any contact with the ball) and a short time limit for practice (5–10 minutes). Samuel is okay with this, and they make a chart on the computer to keep track of the number of swings and the number of hits for each day of practice. Samuel plots the data. He seems to like this plan and his parents see him sometimes go out on his own to practice. He gets confident enough about hitting to play T-ball in the rec program with his friends.

Samuel's parents try a similar plan for a chore, putting the dishes in the dishwasher. Because he dislikes this chore, his parents initially keep the demand small (only his dish and glass) and offer an incentive (points) for each dish/glass beyond this. They increase the demand very gradually and make the incentive easy to earn. Over the course of a month, he is putting the rest of the family dishes in and regularly earning the reward. His parents adopt these approaches as a general strategy to teach Samuel effort and persistence whenever he seems to struggle with an activity or task.

Step 1: Establish Behavioral Goal

Target executive skill(s): Goal-directed persistence

Specific behavioral objective: Samuel will improve his task persistence for preferred and less preferred tasks.

Step 2: Design Intervention

What environmental supports will be provided to help reach the target goal?
- Keep demands easy and establish easily achievable, short goals
- Track progress on a simple chart
- Provide parent support to build the skill

What specific skill will be taught, who will teach the skill, and what procedure will be used to teach it?

Skill: Achievement of goal or completion of task demand through successful completion of small task steps

(cont.)

Who will teach the skill? Samuel's parents will help teach the skill, and Samuel will begin to practice on his own

Procedure:

- Samuel's parents work with him to set achievable goals and task demands.
- Samuel agrees to a practice schedule and criteria.

What incentives will be used to help motivate the child to use/practice the skill?

- Positive feedback indicating that performance objectives are being met
- Charting to make progress visible and concrete
- Points leading to items off reward menu for job completion

👍 **Keys to Success** 👍

- *If your child avoids the activity because he doesn't succeed quickly enough, position the task before a more preferred task.* It's not hard to see that having Samuel do the dishes before he can have computer or TV time might provide an added incentive to do the dishes. But the same may go even for something like practicing batting. The fact that it's a recreational activity doesn't mean practice will seem like fun to a child who has trouble persisting toward a goal. These kids lose their patience quite easily.

Saving Money

From his parents' perspective, 9-year-old Jared is a "here-and-now" type of kid. He doesn't have a lot of patience for waiting and is easily frustrated when he has to work toward a goal or wait for something he wants. For example, he expects to be as good at skateboarding as his best friend even though he started later and doesn't practice as much. Saving the money he gets for allowance or for things like birthdays is especially tough, and as soon as he has money, he wants to go to the store to spend it. As a result he is often broke and routinely asks his parents to either buy him something he wants or to "lend" him the money until he gets his allowance. Getting him to pay the money back can be very difficult, so his parents have adopted a "no loan" policy except in unusual cases. They want to see him learn to follow a plan to get to a future goal, even if it's relatively short-term.

Jared wants a video game system. In the past his parents have told him that he can have one if he saves the money for it. Although he has tried, he hasn't made it past a week or so before he decides to spend his savings on something more immediate. While his parents have concerns about having video games at home, they also see Jared's desire as a means to teach him about getting to a goal. They see Jared potentially working for the system and for the various games he will want. If a savings plan is to work, Jared has to see progress toward his goal fairly quickly. Simply saving the $5 per week that he gets for allowance is not likely to be fast enough. Because his birthday is coming up, the money he gets from his parents, other relatives, and friends can help to "jump start" his fund. Still, his parents know that he needs to see visible progress toward his game system.

His parents decide they will help him develop a plan to buy his game system if he is definitely interested. Talking with him demonstrates that he is. They propose that if Jared is willing to devote all his birthday money toward the game, he could probably buy it in as little as 5 or 6 weeks by adding in his allowance money. Jared is a little uncomfortable with this because it means he will get no presents at his birthday party. He suggests that the four friends he is having over bring birthday presents and he will use the birthday money he gets from his parents and relatives toward the game and then add the rest from allowance. His parents still worry that he will lose sight of the goal. They discuss getting a picture of the game system and laminating it. They will then cut it up into pieces like a puzzle and make each piece correspond to a $5 payment. With his birthday money Jared will get a good start on completing a large part of the puzzle, and then each week another piece will be added with his allowance. Ten weeks after his birthday, Jared completes the puzzle and happily buys his game system. He and his parents like this system and are able to use it for other, longer-term goals.

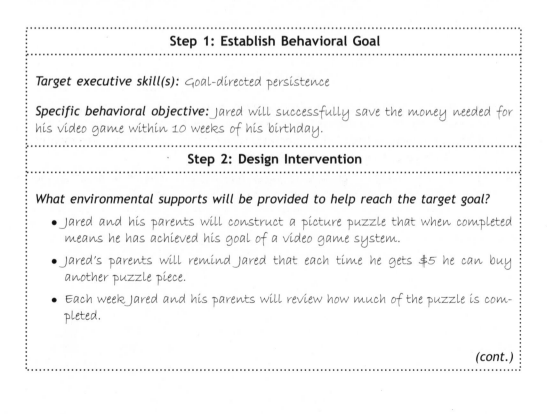

Step 1: Establish Behavioral Goal

Target executive skill(s): Goal-directed persistence

Specific behavioral objective: Jared will successfully save the money needed for his video game within 10 weeks of his birthday.

Step 2: Design Intervention

What environmental supports will be provided to help reach the target goal?

- Jared and his parents will construct a picture puzzle that when completed means he has achieved his goal of a video game system.

- Jared's parents will remind Jared that each time he gets $5 he can buy another puzzle piece.

- Each week Jared and his parents will review how much of the puzzle is completed.

(cont.)

What specific skill will be taught, who will teach the skill, and what procedure will be used to teach it?

Skill: Achievement of a short-term goal through planning and saving

Who will teach the skill? Parents

Procedure:

- Jared and his parents will establish a concrete objective using a picture puzzle.
- Jared's parents will help him set a timeline so that the end is in sight.
- Jared will begin the plan at a time (his birthday) that allows him to get a good jump start on the goal.
- Jared and his parents will formally check the puzzle progress weekly, and his parents will be cheerleaders, encouraging him each time he buys another piece of the puzzle.
- At least every 2 weeks his parents will take Jared to the store to play the demo model of the game so he is in close contact with his goal.

What incentives will be used to help motivate the child to use/practice the skill?

- Jared will have a video game of his own that he otherwise would not have at all.
- Parents will use a similar system for purchase of the games that Jared wants to play.

👍 Keys to Success 👍

- *Remember that a child's time horizon is much shorter than yours.* For a plan like this to succeed, the end always has to be in sight *for the child.* So don't get too ambitious in teaching this skill. Expectations that the child will save for months or put all his resources into savings are unrealistic.

- *Remember that learning to save requires ongoing and long-term practice.* Be prepared to use savings systems over an extended time period.

21

Cultivating Metacognition

Metacognition refers to the ability to stand back and take a bird's-eye view of one-self in a situation. It's an ability to observe how you problem solve. It also includes self-monitoring and self-evaluating—asking yourself, "How am I doing?" or "How did I do?" Adults who have this skill can size up a problem situation, take into account multiple pieces of information, and make good decisions about how to pro-ceed. They can also evaluate afterward how they did and decide to do things differ-ently in the future if need be. Adults who lack this skill may miss or ignore impor-tant information (particularly social cues) and tend to make decisions based on "what feels right" rather than careful analysis of the facts. If you feel like you put your foot in your mouth a lot, make decisions you regret, and can't always get a han-dle on how well you're doing in your endeavors, follow the procedure suggested in Chapter 3 for helping your child learn a skill that isn't your strong suit either.

How Metacognition Develops

Metacognition is a complex set of skills that begins developing during the first year of life as infants work to organize their experiences, by sorting and classifying and by starting to recognize cause–effect relationships. These skills get extended during toddlerhood, when order, routine, and ritual—all mechanisms whereby they can control their experiences—become important to kids. By preschool, the emphasis shifts from exploration to mastery. At this age, children begin to recognize that other people have different perceptual experiences, and they begin to identify emo-tions in others and to be able to role-play. Shortly after that, between the ages of 5 and 7, children begin to recognize that others have different thoughts and feelings, and they start being able to make rudimentary interpretations of intent (such as whether someone hurt them on purpose or by accident). By middle childhood, the metacognitive vista widens dramatically. Children at this age not only have a deeper understanding of their own thoughts, feelings, and intentions, but they understand that their thoughts, feelings, and intentions can be the object of the thinking of others. This is why youngsters in middle school develop such self-consciousness about their own actions and why conformity becomes such a priority for many. They have not yet learned that just because other people *can* think about them in a way that may seem intrusive doesn't mean they are! By high school, they can step back and put things in a little more perspective, as the building blocks of metacognition accumulate and fall into place.

To assess how your child's metacognitive skills compare with his age group, complete the questionnaire below, which builds on the assessment you did of your child in Chapter 2.

HOW WELL DEVELOPED ARE YOUR CHILD'S METACOGNITIVE SKILLS?

Use the following scale to rate how well your child performs each of the tasks listed. At each level, children can be expected to perform all the tasks listed fairly well to very well.

Scale

0—Never or rarely

1—Does but not well (about 25% of the time)

2—Does fairly well (about 75% of the time)

3—Does very well (always or almost always)

Preschool/kindergarten

_____ Can make minor adjustments in a construction project or puzzle task when a first attempt fails

_____ Can come up with a novel (but simple) use of a tool to solve a problem

_____ Makes suggestions to another child for how to fix something

Lower elementary (grades 1-3)

_____ Can adjust behavior in response to feedback from a parent or teacher

_____ Can watch what happens to others and change behavior appropriately

_____ Can verbalize more than one solution to a problem and make the best choice

Upper elementary (grades 4-5)

____ Can anticipate the result of a course of action and make adjustments accordingly (e.g., to avoid getting in trouble)

____ Can articulate several solutions to problems and explain the best one

____ Enjoys the problem-solving component of school assignments or video games

Middle school (grades 6-8)

____ Can accurately evaluate his or her own performance (e.g., in a sports event or school assignment)

____ Can see the impact of his or her behavior on peers and make adjustments (e.g., to fit in with the group or avoid being teased)

____ Can perform tasks requiring more abstract reasoning

Cultivating Metacognitive Skills in Everyday Situations

There are two sets of metacognitive skills that you can help your child develop. One set involves the child's ability to evaluate her performance on a task, such as a chore or a homework assignment, and to make changes based on that evaluation. The second set involves the child's ability to evaluate social situations—both her own behavior and others' reactions and the behavior of others.

To help your child develop skills related to task performance, try the following:

• *Provide specific praise for key elements of task performance.* For instance, if you want to teach your child to be thorough in completing a task, praise him for that: "I like the way you put every single block back in the box" or "I like the way you looked under your bed to see if there were any dirty clothes there."

• *Teach your child to evaluate her own performance on a task.* After finishing her spelling homework where the assignment was to write each spelling word in a sentence, you might ask, "How do you think you did? Did you follow the directions? Do you like the way the paper looks?" You can also offer brief, specific suggestions for improvement, preferably starting with a positive: "You wrote really good sentences, but your words sometimes run together on the page. You might try putting your finger on the page at the end of every word and leaving that much space between one word and the next." In providing feedback and suggestions, suspend judgment because criticism always muddies the water.

• *Have the child identify what finished looks like*. If your son's job is to empty the dishwasher, get him to describe what that means (no more dishes in the dishwasher, everything put away in drawers or cupboards). You may want to write this down and post it prominently to help the child remember.

• *Teach a set of questions children can ask themselves when confronted with problem situations*. These might include: "What is the problem I need to solve?" "What is my plan?" "Am I following my plan?" "How did I do?"

To help your child learn to read social situations, try the following:

• *Play a guessing game to teach your child to read facial expressions*. Many youngsters who have problems with this skill do not know how to read facial expressions or interpret feelings. One way to teach this skill is to turn it into a guessing game where both parents and children make facial expressions and each has to guess what feeling the other person is trying to convey. Another way is to watch a television show with the sound off and guess the person's feelings based on facial expression and body language (you may want to tape the show so that you can rewind and watch segments with the sound on again to check your hypotheses).

• *Help children begin to recognize how tone of voice changes the meaning of what is being said*. It is said that 55% of communication is facial expression, 38% is tone of voice, and only 7% is the actual words spoken. Give your child labels for different tones of voice (teasing, sarcastic, whining, angry) and then ask your child to use them to identify the tones of voice the child uses to communicate as well as those used by others.

• *Talk about the clues to someone's feelings that can be spotted even when the person is trying to hide his feelings*. Are there subtle signs (a tightening of the mouth to signify anger, fiddling with things to denote anxiety)? Turn it into a detective game.

• *Ask your child to identify how her actions might make someone feel*. This teaches the language of feelings and cause–effect relationships.

No More Know-It-All:
Helping Your Child Learn to Listen

Eleven-year-old Yoshi is the oldest of three children in her family. She is a fairly conscientious student. Yoshi has always had a good memory and has always liked to read and watch informative TV like the Discovery channel and *Animal Planet*. As a result of her skills and her interests Yoshi has stored a lot of information and has become something of a "junior expert" on a variety of subjects. Her parents and her relatives have encouraged this and continue to look to her for information at times. Yoshi likes to share her wealth of information with others, enjoying the role of expert and the praise she sometimes gets from adults. But she doesn't know where to draw the line. She often corrects others or dismisses what they have to say, dominating the conversation. At home, this has become a major source of conflict with her two younger siblings. Her parents now see that Yoshi's volunteering the knowledge she's gained is a problem at times. Yoshi's closest friends are tiring of her being a know-it-all, and in school this behavior has caused conflicts in the classroom. For her part, Yoshi is sometimes aware of people's reactions to her comments or corrections, but she tends to see it as their issue, not hers. Yoshi's parents are concerned about the rift her behavior is creating in the family and between their daughter and her peers.

When her parents initially approach her, Yoshi insists that she isn't doing anything "wrong" and that she is trying to be helpful to other people. But as they talk more, Yoshi admits that she is worried because sometimes she feels that people don't like her.

Helping Yoshi is complicated because talking about what she knows is so automatic. Yoshi suggests that maybe they can start working on this at home because it happens often with her siblings, especially at family meals. Her parents suggest and she agrees that the first step is to think about being a listener rather than a talker. The second step, for now, is accepting what people say and not correcting them.

To start the plan, Yoshi agrees to practice being a "listener" by being the last person at the table to speak, after her siblings and parents have spoken. When she does speak, she can ask them for more information about their topic and/or compliment them. She also can talk about her activities and interests. Yoshi and her parents have worked out a cueing system so that if she begins to correct or "lecture," they can signal her. Before starting, the family gets together and Yoshi explains how she is trying to change and what she will do.

At first Yoshi finds it difficult to follow the plan and often sits through meals silently. Over time, however, with her parents modeling compliments and questions, she is able to do this herself and interact without giving corrections or advice. She begins using the same strategies with her friends and with peers in school. She is comfortable enough to tell her teacher about her plan, and her teacher agrees to cue her if she begins to dominate a discussion or criticize others. Because she is not always being a know-it-all, adults and peers are more inclined to ask her for opinions and information.

Step 1: Establish Behavioral Goal

Target executive skill(s): Metacognition

Specific behavioral objective: To increase listening and decrease lecturing and correcting others in conversations

(cont.)

Step 2: Design Intervention

What environmental supports will be provided to help reach the target goal?

- Other people in the family will speak first.
- Parents/teacher will cue Yoshi if she begins to lecture or correct.
- Parents/teacher model listening and acceptable conversation behaviors.

What specific skill will be taught, who will teach the skill, and what procedure will be used to teach it?

Skill: In a social interaction, listening before speaking and demonstrating interest in what others have to say

Who will teach the skill? Parents/teacher/friends

Procedure:

- Yoshi is the last person to speak at family meals.
- Yoshi's comments are directed at getting additional information from the listener or complimenting what the listener says.
- Parents cue lecturing or correcting.
- Yoshi models parents' verbal behavior.
- Yoshi tries these techniques at school and with friends.

What incentives will be used to help motivate the child to use/practice the skill?

- Parents and teacher compliment Yoshi on her listening skills.
- Friends welcome Yoshi into the group and negative comments stop.

👍 Keys to Success 👍

- *Because you can't always be on hand to monitor your child's behavior, you'll need an alternative to keep track of progress.* One possibility is to have your child keep track (even informally) of situations when she has listened to her siblings or friends without interrupting or correcting and report back to you, giving a few specific examples. Another possibility is for the child to arrange with one trusted friend to give her a subtle cue if she starts to dominate.

- *When helping your child evaluate his performance, keep in mind that what's important to you is not always important to your child.* The best way to handle this may be to agree to meet in the middle. The standard to be working toward should not be perfection, but a degree of quality that the child can feel good about. Just as adults will choose to put more time and effort into some tasks than others, children need to be allowed to do this as well—not every homework assignment will be a masterpiece, not every social interaction a triumph.

Learning to Evaluate Performance

Cory is 14, an eighth grader with a 10-year-old sister. The two live primarily with their mother and see their father one night during the week and on alternate weekends. Mom works full-time, and the children are expected to share chores around the house. In addition, Cory takes care of his sister some days after school. He plays the trumpet in the band and works about 10 hours a week in a local grocery store, retrieving grocery carts.

Cory sees himself as motivated and fairly hard working, but he's an average student. Since entering middle school he's been increasingly frustrated about what he feels is a lack of payoff for the amount of work he puts in. In school his grades don't seem to reflect the fact that he does his homework without needing to be reminded or prodded and studies for tests. At work he is reliable, but he hasn't had a raise since he started, and his manager sometimes says he needs to be more attentive. At home he carries out his chores and is more than willing to help out. Since he was young, however, his mother has always had to check on his work and at times have him complete or redo a task that he thought he had finished.

Cory's weakness has always been in checking his work. When he was young this was less of an issue because his parents or teachers were there to monitor him closely. But now that he's older he's expected to review his work more independently. Cory's mother gives him concrete examples of where his inconsistency affects the quality of his work, from spotty vacuuming to failing to edit essays assigned at school. Cory has always been willing to accept such feedback and correct his work, so what he needs to do is figure out in advance what needs to be checked so he can monitor rather than waiting for other people to tell him his work hasn't measured up after he's completed it.

Using vacuuming as an example, his mother asks Cory to think about the task and create a "start-to-finish" list for what would be a thorough job. When he is done they look at the list together and his mother suggests one additional step. This becomes Cory's list for this chore. Understanding the idea, Cory goes to his manager and asks how he could improve his performance on his specific job. His manager is happy to oblige, and Cory arranges to check back with him in 2 weeks to see if he has it right. School is a little more complicated because of the number of subjects and the variety of work. Cory and his mother first meet with his teaching team, and he explains what he wants to work on. Together they review his report cards and progress reports to see if there are specific areas where the problem is more likely to come up. From this information the teachers see that writing assignments are the primary problem. His English teacher suggests that they meet because this is her area. She provides a task list (rubric) for his writing assignments, and she agrees to review this with Cory prior to his starting an assignment and also to look at Cory's first draft to determine how well he has monitored his work and followed the rubric. Having the lists in these different areas, reviewing them beforehand, and having someone (teacher, manager, etc.) evaluate his monitoring helps Cory improve his work. From this process, he realizes that when he gets feedback that he needs to be more careful or thorough, he will need to follow a similar plan for the task or job.

Step 1: Establish Behavioral Goal

Target executive skill(s): Metacognition

Specific behavioral objective: During specific tasks, Cory will evaluate his performance against a standard given for that task and work to meet the standard.

Step 2: Design Intervention

What environmental supports will be provided to help reach the target goal?

- Parent/manager/teacher provide standards (in list form) for selected tasks in each of their areas
- Parent/manager/teacher provide feedback about performance to Cory

What specific skill will be taught, who will teach the skill, and what procedure will be used to teach it?

Skill: Cory will learn to evaluate and, where needed, correct his performance so that it meets a standard given for that task.

Who will teach the skill? Parent/manager/teacher will provide standard and performance feedback.

Procedure:

- Cory, together with adults, chooses a set of tasks for monitoring and improvement.
- Adults provide an acceptable performance standard for these tasks.
- Cory reviews expectations before beginning the task.
- Cory performs tasks, monitors performance, and adults provide feedback on how well the standard was met.
- Cory corrects his performance as needed.

What incentives will be used to help motivate the child to use/practice the skill?

- Positive feedback from adults about performance
- Improved grades in school and improved job performance leading to raises

👍 Keys to Success 👍

- *Don't try to tackle too many different behaviors at once.* Limit the intervention to one or two in the beginning. It's probably also best to address only one domain at a time, such as home or school, not both.

- *Give your child very specific feedback about very specific behaviors to be changed.* This plan has a good chance of succeeding if your child is motivated and can accept feedback from others, but even then it's doomed to fail if you say things like "You need to be more careful," your child's teacher says, "Spend more time studying," or the child's boss says, "Pay attention when you're working." Your child needs concrete directions such as "Check all six rows between the cars for shopping carts as well as the return areas."

22

··

When What You Do Is Not Enough

For children with significant executive skill weaknesses, what you can do on your own to resolve the problem may very well prove insufficient. If you've tried the strategies and suggestions presented so far in this book with little success, and the troubleshooting advice offered in Chapters 11–21 hasn't helped, you need to look a little more closely at what's going on.

When a home plan is not working, we suggest you take a close look at the intervention to make sure the key elements necessary for success are in place. As we've said, and hopefully demonstrated, you *can* improve your child's executive skills. As we have also said, doing so involves effort and attention to detail, especially on the front end of the plan. Although it may seem simplistic, it is important to quickly review each step of the plan.

If you came to us, these are the questions we would ask:

What is the specific problem you've attempted to tackle? For example, does your child cry with any change in plans? Does she have to spend money as soon as she gets it? Does he lose or misplace belongings on a daily basis? Have you stated the problem definition with enough specificity to enable you to judge success or failure? The description of the behavior needs to be precise enough so that you, your child, and anyone else involved has no doubt about whether the behavior has occurred. Descriptions that include the words *always, never, everything, all the time,* and *so forth* are likely to be too general. For example, "Kim is constantly losing her belongings," "Jack is late for everything," "Mikey cries at the drop of a hat," "Amy is late all the time," and "Tyler can't follow directions" do not provide sufficient information either to address the problem or to evaluate the success of the plan. Specifying what (for example, what does she lose), when (at what times is the behavior most likely or does it pose the biggest problem), and where (in what situations does it happen most) helps better define the problem. Even if the behavior happens across more situations, the key is to pick a specific starting point (remember, "baby steps").

What is your standard for judging that the problem has improved and what behavior can you live with? Wholesale behavior change is not only hard to elicit but may be well-nigh impossible, at least in the short term, so we encourage you to be realistic in your expectations for improvement. List two or three specific situations where the problem occurs now, state how you want things to go in those situations, and state what you would like your child to do. Some examples: (1) voices displeasure with change but accepts it without tantrum; (2) saves at least 30% of any money earned; (3) requires your help to find missing materials no more than twice a week. It's important to start with small improvements and build on these rather than expecting that the problem will be completely resolved. Baby steps toward the goal should be considered a success.

Given your child's age, current skills, and the amount of effort needed from your child to accomplish what you want, are your expectations realistic? Watch how you answer this question. If you find yourself saying, with some exasperation, "When I was her age I certainly didn't have this problem" or "Every other kid his age can handle this situation without falling apart," you may be reaching too high. Go back to the previous question: what can you live with as evidence of improvement?

What environmental supports have you put in place? For example, do you have a visual cue to signal that a change in plans is coming? When your child receives money, is a place to store it immediately available? Do storage spaces for belongings have specific pictures or written labels?

What specific skill are you trying to teach? As with the problem definition, you need to be clear about the behavior you are trying to teach. Although we've encouraged you to begin by identifying the executive skill involved, these skills are taught in the context of more specific behaviors. In the examples above, you may be teaching your child to recognize and react acceptably to a change symbol, to take the money she's earned and immediately put it in her bank, or to place toys in a specific storage area.

Who is responsible for teaching the skill, what is the procedure, and how often is it done/practiced? Particularly in the beginning stages of helping your child improve executive skills, the burden is as much on the person teaching the skill as it is on the child. Our job as parents would be so much easier if what psychologists call *one-trial learning* worked for the skills we wanted our kids to acquire. In reality, most of the important behaviors we expect children to master by the time they leave our homes require practice over a long period of time. Have you built that into your plan?

What incentives are being used to help motivate your child to learn the new skill/behavior and practice it when the situation arises? We've found that it is often this step that is missing in the plan. Rewards that your child values can be a powerful incentive to get the child to try the plan to begin with and then as a way to signal success. Once the child learns the skill, natural incentives such as your approval and praise can be enough to maintain the skill. We do not look at rewards as "bribes," but some parents are uncomfortable using them. If you're among them, use one of your child's preferred activities and make access to this activity contingent on demonstration of the behavior you want.

If you believe you've addressed these issues and developed a reasonable, specific plan with supports and incentives, there are still a few other factors to consider when a plan is not working.

- *The consistency with which the plan is followed.* We're all busy, and it's not always easy or convenient to make sure your child has been cued about a schedule change or monitored to ensure that money or belongings are stored away. Incentives are not always given in a timely fashion. Occasional slip-ups are bound to happen, and they will not cause a plan to fail. On the other hand, if the plan is followed only intermittently, it *will* fail. You'll see that your child is not changing, and therefore there is little incentive for you to work at the plan. Your child will see that the plan is not important to you, and hence will make less effort, returning instead to old behaviors. For these reasons, plans should be relatively simple and fit within the time frames that you reliably have available.

- *Consistency among adults using the plan.* If another parent, an older sibling, or a teacher is supposed to use the plan or some part of it, he or she must adhere to the key elements or the plan is likely to fail. A mother we know wanted to implement a savings plan using allowance, but her husband initially resisted because he hadn't received an allowance as a child and did not think his children should. The mother put the plan on hold until she sold him on the benefits of their child learning to save for a future goal. Had she implemented the plan without him, problems were likely. If several people share child care/management responsibilities, they should discuss the plan and agree on the role each will play from the beginning. If the plan involves homework or school materials (books, etc.), parents and teachers should be clear about what is expected from each, the frequency of communication and how this will occur, and in most cases, the method of communication should not involve the child, since children are notoriously poor informants.

- *The time that the plan is in place.* There are no hard-and-fast rules about how long a plan should be tried. If the plan is reasonable—that is, it meets most of the preceding criteria—try it for 14 to 21 days. This may not seem long, but in our experience parents typically try a plan for 4–5 days and then become inconsistent. You too may fall prey to this temptation, for two reasons: If you don't see any change, the lack of immediate payoff may make it difficult to sustain the necessary effort. On the other hand, you may see an almost immediate improvement, feel like you've accomplished what you hoped for, and slack off. In this case, the change does not last, and within a few weeks the old pattern returns. To keep yourself honest, you may want to take time at the end of each day the plan is in place to rate how well you stuck to the plan, using a 5-point scale (1, *I really screwed up today*, to 5, *I stuck to the plan 100%!*).

How do I know whether my child can't or won't? Maybe she is just lazy!

In all our years of professional practice, we have met very few children we would call lazy. We've met children who are discouraged, who doubt their abilities, who feel it is more punishing to try and fail than not try at all, or who prefer to spend time doing things they find fun rather than things they find tedious or difficult. The critical issue is not whether children can't or won't, but what it would take to help them overcome whatever obstacle is preventing them from acquiring proficiency at tasks or completing tasks that are currently not getting done. The way to help them overcome obstacles usually involves a combination of modifying the task so it doesn't seem so daunting, teaching them the steps to follow to complete the task and supervising them as they do it, and building in an incentive to make it worth their while to engage in work that feels effortful to them. If you do all this, they can be smart but not scattered.

Seeking Professional Help

So you've done the best you can, and you're still not seeing much improvement. Now what? It's certainly true that some children have more challenging executive skill problems than parents can handle easily on their own. If you decide your child is one of these children, you can look for help from a licensed clinician such as a psychologist, social worker, or mental health counselor. The title of the professional is less important than the orientation of the clinician's practice. We recommend finding a specialist who uses either a behavioral or a cognitive-behavioral approach and is experienced in parent training.

Clinicians who use a behavioral approach focus on identifying the specific environmental triggers that contribute to the problem behavior (called *antecedents*) as well as the way behavior is responded to (called *consequences*). They then help parents alter either the antecedents or the consequences or both. Cognitive-behavioral therapists may use a similar approach, but they also address how children and their parents *think* about the problem situations and teach them to think differently (for example, by giving them coping strategies such as self-talk, relaxation strategies, and thought-stopping techniques). We do not recommend therapists who use traditional talk therapy or relationship therapy, because we believe that children and their parents benefit from learning specific skills and strategies for handling problems caused by weak executive skills.

When Testing Might Be Warranted

Parents of children with more severe executive skill problems often ask us if they should have their child tested. We are not big advocates of testing as a way to identify executive skill weaknesses because the tests that have been developed to assess executive skills often do not correlate well with what parents and teachers know about the child being assessed. Nonetheless, those situations in which testing may be useful include:

- If you think your child will need additional support in school, for which an evaluation might provide the necessary documentation that there is a problem that needs to be addressed.
- If you think there may be additional learning problems (such as a learning disability or an attention disorder) that an evaluation could help clarify.
- If you think there may be other explanations for the behavior of concern that may suggest different treatment options. Psychological disorders such as bipolar disorder, anxiety, depression, and obsessive–compulsive disorders all have an impact on executive skills. There are treatments that have been developed to treat disorders such as these (including medication and specific therapeutic approaches), and an accurate diagnosis would be helpful in pointing you in the direction of an appropriate intervention.

If you decide to seek an evaluation that would include an assessment of your child's executive skill strengths and weaknesses, the professionals that typically do this kind of assessment include psychologists, neuropsychologists, and school psychologists. If the problems are significant enough to cause school failure, then schools are obligated to provide this kind of evaluation. (See the next chapter for further clarification about what constitutes school failure.)

In addition to whatever "tests" the evaluator might use (such as IQ tests or achievement tests), the specialist should use rating scales designed to assess executive skills (such as the Behavior Rating Inventory of Executive Function, or BRIEF) as well as collect information, usually through a detailed interview, from parents about how the executive skill problems show up in the everyday life of the child. The benefit of collecting this kind of information is that it leads naturally to the development of interventions, which is, after all, the primary purpose of an evaluation.

Thoughts on Medication

Medications are used to treat psychological disorders or biologically based disorders such as ADHD, anxiety disorders, and obsessive–compulsive disorders. These medications may result in improvement in executive functioning, but they were not designed specifically for that purpose.

Stimulant medications have been shown in many studies conducted over many years to be very effective in controlling a number of the symptoms associated with ADHD, including distractibility, difficulty completing work, overactivity, and impulse control. Because children with ADHD can work more efficiently and persist longer with tasks when they take stimulants, improvements with time management and goal-directed persistence may be seen. Medications for anxiety disorders can address problems with emotional control when those problems are due to underlying anxiety. We know of no studies that have pinpointed specific executive skills to determine whether the use of medication leads to improvement either in the executive skill itself or in tasks that require the use of specific executive skills.

The parents we see in our clinical practice usually prefer to try nonmedical interventions first, and we support this approach. The use of medication may lead parents and teachers to believe that this intervention alone is sufficient, and we believe the effectiveness of medication can be enhanced when it is combined with behavioral or psychosocial interventions. Furthermore, some research studies suggest that when medication is combined with other interventions, lower dosages can be prescribed. For these reasons, we recommend using approaches such as environmental modifications, home-school report cards, and incentive systems prior to considering medication.

There may be times, however, when medication use is warranted. For children with ADHD, there are a number of warning signs parents may look for that signal that a trial of stimulant medication might be worth considering. These include:

- *When the attention disorder (especially impulsivity and motor activity level) is having an impact on a child's ability to make or keep friends.* The ability to form social relationships in childhood is a strong predictor of good adjustment throughout life, and if attention problems prevent this from happening, medication may be warranted.
- *When the attention disorder begins to affect self-esteem.* Children with even milder forms of ADHD become aware that their attention problems are making them stand out in school (for example, the teacher is always prompting them to pay attention) or are preventing them from achieving success in schoolwork (for example, by leading them to make many careless mistakes). When children start making negative comments about themselves, the attention disorder is likely having an impact on self-esteem that may be reduced through the use of medication.
- *When the attention disorder interferes directly with the child's ability to learn.* This can happen in several ways: (1) they have difficulty sustaining attention in class and therefore miss instruction or fail to complete seatwork; (2) they become so easily frustrated that they give up and learning becomes short-circuited; or (3) they lack the patience to plan and execute tasks that can't be done quickly. This is seen either in a child's difficulty *slowing down* when tasks require this for success or in an inability to handle multistep problems because they lack the capacity to think through the steps involved to achieve success.
- *When the amount of effort required on the part of the child to control his*

distractibility, impulsivity, or motor activity is great enough to affect his overall level of emotional adjustment.

For youngsters for whom emotional control is problematic, due to either depression or anxiety, parents should consider the severity of the problem when making medication decisions. Research with adults suggests that cognitive-behavioral therapy may be just as effective in treating anxiety and depression as is medication, but when this kind of therapy is unavailable, and the child's depression or anxiety is pervasive enough to significantly affect quality of life, medication is worth considering.

23

Working with the School

Children with weak executive skills not only have problems at home. They also have problems in school, and in fact it's often the school problems that bring parents to our office. What's frustrating for many of the parents we work with is that they can work really hard at home to address the problems, but they have no control over the school environment and the problems that arise there. This book would not be complete if it didn't offer advice and guidance on how to work with schools.

Here's what we've learned from years of working on executive skill problems with parents, teachers, and students: for genuine improvement to occur, *everybody has to work harder.* Teachers have to do more for children with executive skill weaknesses than for other students, you need to provide more supervision and monitoring than a typical child would need, and children with executive skill weaknesses will have to work harder than they would have to if all their executive skills were developing normally. We have found that tensions, conflict, and unhappiness are most likely to occur if any one of these three parties is not pulling his or her weight.

Tactically, a nonadversarial approach usually works better than blame or accusations in persuading teachers to change how they handle a child. Working from the premise that everyone has to work harder, we generally recommend that you start the conversation with your child's teacher by laying out the problem as you see it and saying, "Here's what we can do, and here's what we're prepared to ask our child to do." Follow this with an open-ended question, such as "What do you think would help?" For example, for a child who has trouble getting all his homework done and remembering to hand it in, you might say, "We're willing to check his assignment book every night, make a homework plan with him, and supervise him to make sure he's put his homework in a homework folder and the homework folder in his backpack. What else can be done to make sure the homework actually gets handed in?" If your child's teacher doesn't feel that it's his or her responsibility to provide any individual support to address the problem, you may want to refer the teacher to this book or the one we wrote specifically for educators (*Executive Skills in Children and*

Adolescents: A Practical Guide to Assessment and Intervention). This will give the teacher a better understanding of executive skills and ideas for how to address the problem in the classroom.

Here are some of the school-related issues that frequently arise in our work with parents:

My daughter's teacher clearly thinks that if my daughter were on medication, everyone would be a lot happier. I'd prefer to try other things first. How can I handle this? Our response to this question is straightforward: Medication should never be a school decision. Rather, medication decisions are exclusively an issue between you and your child's physician. It may be easier for teachers or other educators to accept your response to their raising medication as a possibility if you couch it in terms of your hesitation about medication. You might say, "I'm nervous about my child taking medication. I know there can be side effects, and that worries me. Here's what I would like to try . . . " If you let teachers know you're willing to try harder, they may be more willing to try harder, too.

My child's teacher says he'll make accommodations for my child's executive skill problems (like checking in with him at the end of the day to make sure he has everything he needs for homework or sending home a weekly progress report so I can find out about missing assignments), but then he forgets to do it and my son fails assignments as a result. What can I do about this? If the teacher is well intentioned (but perhaps has executive skill weaknesses of his own), you should be sympathetic. "I know you're busy at the end of the day. Is there something I could do to help?" Some teachers only grudgingly agree to provide increased cueing, monitoring, or supervision, however, and when they fall short, the truth comes out. "I think your child should be doing this himself," they may say when pressed. The response to this kind of comment is "We've tried that before and it hasn't been effective. We need to do something more than hold him accountable to do this all on his own." There are things you can do to make it easier for teachers, though. We often recommend that parents email teachers on a weekly basis to find out about missing homework assignments. Because it's easier to reply to an email than to generate one, this reduces the burden on the teacher and may make the communication task more manageable. We've also known mothers who have happily come to their child's school once a week to help clean out desks or lockers. In neither case are parents or teachers letting the child "off the hook." Rather, they're putting in place systems that help hold children accountable while supervising them at the same time.

What is reasonable to expect classroom teachers to do to help my child develop more effective executive skills? We've found that those teachers who are most effective in supporting the development of executive skills are ones who create whole-class routines that help children develop skills such as organization, planning, working memory, and time management. They also embed instruction in executive skills into subject matter teaching. They teach children how to break down long-term assignments into subtasks and to develop timelines for subtask completion. They build in homework routines to ensure that students remember to hand in their homework and end-of-day routines to help children learn to check their assignment books and put in their backpacks everything they need for homework. They develop classroom rules for behavior that help children control impulses and manage their emotions, and they review the rules regularly and at opportune times (for example, just before a guest is about to address the class or just before recess).

Again, because teachers like everyone else have executive skill strengths and weaknesses, some teachers incorporate these kinds of activities more than others. If your child has a teacher who doesn't do this well, it's reasonable to look for resources other than the teacher to help—a classroom aide, guidance counselor, principal or assistant principal, etc. Many schools offer Teacher Assistance Teams where classroom teachers, administrators, and specialists meet regularly to discuss how to address learning or behavior problems of specific students. You can ask that your child be put on that agenda and meet with the team to brainstorm solutions to the problem.

When are executive skill problems severe enough to warrant additional services, such as a Section 504 Plan or special education? How do I access those services? The general rule of thumb we subscribe to is that when a child's executive skill weaknesses interfere with that child's ability to succeed in school, additional services are warranted. Certainly, failing grades would be evidence of school failure. But we would also argue that grades that don't reflect a child's potential when those poor grades attributed to executive skill weaknesses also signal a need for additional supports. These supports might be provided informally (as implied in the answer to the previous question), but they also may be provided more formally, either through a Section 504 Plan or through special education.

504 Plans and special education are governed by laws and regulations that specify who is eligible for services and for what kinds of services. Section 504 is a civil rights law that prohibits discrimination against individuals with disabilities. It's designed to ensure that children with disabilities have access to the same education that children without disabilities have access to. The services provided under this law are typically accommodations and modifications provided in the regular classroom and designed to enable the child to benefit from classroom instruction. Examples of these include allowing extended time on tests or alternative test methods, modified homework assignments, allowing for breaks (so a child with ADHD, for instance, can get up and move around or leave the classroom temporarily), and modified grading procedures (for example, weighing daily work higher than tests if the student tests poorly).

Special education is intended for children with an educational disability that adversely affects educational performance and that requires specialized instruction to correct. Children with executive skill deficits may qualify for a 504 Plan to build appropriate modifications or accommodations into the classroom, or they may qualify for special education when direct instruction is needed. Helping a student learn to become organized, to manage time effectively, or to do the planning required to complete long-term projects or to juggle multiple assignments at once very often requires individualized instruction that would warrant special education. In either case, begin with your child's teacher and ask how to contact the 504 coordinator or special education coordinator for the building. Request that a meeting be set up where your child's problems can be discussed and steps can be taken to determine whether the child is eligible for either special education or a 504 Plan.

Special education has traditionally involved a comprehensive evaluation to determine whether the child has an educational disability that would qualify him for special education services. The most common disabilities are learning disabilities, emotional or behavioral disorders, a speech/language handicap, mental impairment or mental retardation, or another health impairment (referred to as OHI, or other health impaired), such as ADHD or another medical condition that might affect learning. However, in the most recent revision of the federal special education laws, states and local schools now have the option of using a response-to-intervention model, or RTI. This is an assessment–intervention model that begins with high-quality instruction and behavioral supports in the regular classroom. When children struggle in that setting, a series of interventions are put in place to address the problem, beginning with fine-tuning classroom-based interventions and increasing in intensity as necessary to address the problem. This model emphasizes high-quality instruction as well as data-based decision making so that there will be no question of the success of any intervention attempted.

We think this approach lends itself well to the needs of children with executive skill deficits. For instance, let's say Kevin, age 15, is failing geometry because he is handing in only 50% of his homework assignments. His test grades are good, in part because he actually does most of his homework, but he loses it or forgets to hand it in about half the time. The obvious first step to help Kevin (who clearly has problems with organization and working memory!) is to design systems to prevent him from losing his homework and to cue him in class to help him remember to hand in his homework. Under the traditional special education framework, Kevin's parents—or even his math teacher—might refer him to special education for an evaluation to determine whether he has a disability. With an RTI model, Kevin and his parents and teacher could meet and design an intervention they think will work. Using the principle that *everyone has to work harder*, Kevin's parents could agree to check in with Kevin each night before he goes to bed to make sure he has put his geometry homework in a folder designated for that purpose (Kevin decides a fluorescent green folder picked up from a local office supply store will do nicely). If he has remembered to put the assignment in his folder without a reminder from his parents, he'll earn points from his parents, which he can use to save up for a video game he wants to purchase. His geometry teacher agrees to institute a procedure whereby he collects the homework assignments from each student individually as soon as the class has finished the homework review. If these steps are successful in resolving the problem, and there's no reason to believe they won't be, assuming each person involved in the intervention plays her part consistently, then there's no need to go further in the special education process.

For another student, however, who fails to hand in his homework because he doesn't understand the material, a different intervention will need to be designed, and this one may lead to the need for special education services.

I think my child needs to be on an IEP (Individualized Education Plan). How would you write an IEP for someone with executive skill weaknesses? Based on the most recent revision of the federal special education laws (the Individuals with Disabilities Education Improvement Act, or IDEIA), IEPs must include measurable annual goals and a statement about how progress will be measured. For a student with executive skill deficits, an IEP should include a description of the specific skill to be addressed as well as how it manifests itself in the classroom or on specific academic tasks. The method of measurement is tied to the functional behavior and should be as objective as possible. Progress can be measured by (1) counting behaviors (for example, the number of times a child gets in a fight on the playground); (2) calculating a percentage (for example, percent of homework handed in on time); (3) rating performance using a rating scale with each point on the rating scale carefully defined; or (4) using naturally occurring data such as test or quiz scores, absences from class, number of discipline referrals, etc.

An example for a student who has difficulty completing class assignments because he's slow to get started and has difficulty sticking with the task long enough to get it done is shown below.

Sample Task Initiation/Sustained Attention IEP Goals

Goal 1	Student will complete class assignments within the time frame set by the teacher.
How goals will be measured	Teacher will count percentage of assignments finished within the allotted time. Results will be graphed by student and teacher at the end of each day.
Goal 2	Student will start all classroom assignments within 5 minutes of designated start time.
How goal will be measured	Teacher will set kitchen timer at the designated start time. When the bell rings, teacher checks with student to see if the assignment has been started. Percent of assignments started on time will be graphed by student and teacher at the end of each day.

My child has an IEP (or 504 Plan) with executive skill goals, but the school is not following it. What can I do to get them to do what they say they will do? The first step is to make sure that the goals and measurement procedures are defined precisely. This includes stating the IEP goal in measurable terms and defining not only *how* the goal will be measured but also when and by whom (see the examples above). If this is in place, you can then ask the IEP team to share the data with you whenever they collect the data or on a regular basis (for example, weekly, biweekly, monthly). As much as possible, we recommend that data be kept on a computer (such as on a spreadsheet) so that results can be emailed easily to you. You may want to ask your child's case manager if it would make it easier for he or she to remember to share the data with you if you send email reminders at the appropriate times.

Creating IEP goals that are precise and measurable is a relatively new venture for schools. This, combined with the fact that teachers may not have experience writing IEP goals to address executive skill deficits, means that you may need to be patient with schools and to offer assistance—for example, by sharing the sample goals in the table on pages 294–296.

As we stated earlier, you're likely to get more cooperation, and therefore better results, when you take a nonadversarial approach with schools. However, if, despite your best efforts, you hit a dead end in your efforts to collaborate with your child's teacher or special education team, you may have no recourse but to hire an advocate or a lawyer to help you get the services your child needs.

Sample IEP Goals and Measurement Procedures

Executive skill	Sample annual goal	How progress will be measured
Response inhibition	In class discussions, student will raise his hand and wait to be called on 90% of the time before giving an oral response.	Teacher will compute percentage of "hand-raising" responses given over total number of responses given. Student and teacher will graph results weekly.
Working memory	Student will hand in all homework assignments on time.	Teacher will compute percentage of homework handed in on time each week; results will be entered in a graphing program and emailed to student and his parents every Friday.
Emotional control	Student will maintain self-control when given assignments she finds frustrating.	Teacher will keep running tally of "meltdowns" during independent work time; graph will be completed weekly and shared with student every Friday.

Executive skill	Sample annual goal	How progress will be measured
Sustained attention	Student will complete class assignments within time frame set by teacher.	Teacher will count percentage of assignments finished within allotted time; student and teacher will keep daily graph of results.
Task initiation	Student will start all classroom assignments within 5 minutes of designated start time.	Teacher will set kitchen timer at designated start time. When the bell rings, will check in with student to see if the assignment is begun. Percent of assignments started on time will be graphed by student and teacher daily.
Planning/ prioritization	With teacher supervision, student will complete project planning form for every long-term assignment, including a description of steps or subtasks and timelines for each item.	Teacher will review project planning form and with student grade quality of planning description using a 1-5 scale (1 = *poorly planned with missing elements or unrealistic/ unspecified timelines*, 5 = *well planned, all critical elements defined with precision, complete and realistic time lines*); scores will be maintained on a running graph.
Organization	Student will maintain neat desk in the classroom with places allocated for books, notebooks, pencils, etc., and no extraneous materials.	Student and teacher will write a list of what a neat desk looks like. Teacher will conduct random spot checks at least once a week, and together student and teacher will judge how many items on the list are present. Results will be maintained on a running graph.
Time management	Student will estimate correctly how long it takes to complete daily homework assignments and will make and follow a homework schedule.	Student will write a daily plan listing all work to be completed, an estimate of how long each task will take, and start and stop times for each task. Coach and student will review previous day's plan every day and rate how well the plan was followed using a 1-5 scale (1 = *poorly developed plan, poorly executed*, 5 = *well-developed plan, followed successfully, with accurate time estimates for task completion*). Results will be maintained on a running graph.

(cont.)

Executive skill	Sample annual goal	How progress will be measured
Goal-directed persistence	With assistance from guidance counselor, student will complete college application process, applying to at least four schools and getting applications in by deadline.	Student and guidance counselor will create a plan for completing college application process, with deadlines for each step in plan. Guidance counselor will track number of cues or reminders needed for student to complete each step in plan; results will be graphed and shared with student on a weekly basis.
Flexibility	Student will use coping strategies to get back on track when he meets obstacles in completing class assignments.	Student will complete coping strategies checklist; teacher will track percentage of time he returns to his work within 5 minutes.

24

....

What's Ahead?

Mark Twain once said, "As a boy of 14, my father was so ignorant I could hardly stand to have the old man around. But when I got to be 21, I was astonished at how much he had learned in seven years." We have chosen in this book to cover children through the lower end of Mark Twain's range, but no doubt you have some questions about what to expect as your child ventures further into adolescence and out the other end into adulthood.

Several factors conspire to make it challenging for parents and youngsters to manage demands on executive skills during the teenage years. At this age, particularly in middle school and early in high school, conformity is more important than at any age earlier or later. Youngsters at this age yearn to be "normal" or just like everyone else, and they tend to resist any notion that there might be some aspect of their functioning that isn't working well. The peer group becomes far more important than parents at this age in terms of influencing attitudes and motivations. Youngsters at this age are also developing a far greater capacity to think abstractly; one of the ways they "practice" this newfound skill is through "argumentation," and they seem particularly to enjoy practicing this skill with parents. This may be because another major developmental task of this period is to assert one's independence from parents. When this is combined with the adolescent conceit that one knows far more than one's parents, this age can become particularly challenging for parents. The Mark Twain quote exemplifies this attitude. It's difficult to preach patience to parents of early adolescents, but things do improve with maturity.

Another reason that teenagers with executive skill weaknesses often struggle more than ever is because the demands placed on executive skills become greater. By the time youngsters reach middle school and high school, they're expected to work independently, to keep track of more complex assignments and responsibilities, and to plan and execute long-term assignments such as studying for exams and completing multistep projects. At the same time this is happening, the supports that parents and teachers provide to younger children tend to fall away around the mid-

297

dle school years because it's assumed that students at this age can handle the responsibility on their own.

Teenagers also begin to resist the kinds of supports and supervision that benefited them when they were younger. This, too, is consistent with the major developmental task of achieving independence and breaking away from adult authority figures. And finally, teenagers have available to them a large number of interests and activities that compete for their time. Hanging out with friends, playing video games, surfing the net or IMing all are more attractive to teenagers than doing homework. Youngsters with executive skill weaknesses often have a "good enough" mentality when they approach their studies anyway. This becomes accentuated when there's an array of more attractive activities before them.

All this may be a reasonable argument to work with your child to improve on address executive skill problems before the child becomes too firmly entrenched in all the developmental tasks that define this developmental period. If you find yourself approaching your child's freshman year in high school with far more trepidation than he is, here are some developmentally appropriate strategies you should consider:

- *Use natural or logical consequences.* A natural consequence of failing to complete homework assignments during the week is having to catch up on weekends. A logical consequence is that you lose the chance to hang out with friends on Saturday night because the time is needed for studying.
- *Make access to privileges contingent on performance.* Once kids learn to drive, access to the family car becomes a powerful incentive. And all those electronics that teenagers crave can be earned over time and accessible contingently.
- *Be willing to negotiate and make deals.* Inflexible parents—as well as those who have strong misgivings about the use of incentives—deprive themselves of powerful motivators to help kids develop more effective executive skills.
- *Work on positive communication skills.* Nothing derails a conversation with a teenager faster than putdowns, sarcasm, and not listening to other points of view (even when your child is engaging in the same communication patterns). See the table below for a list of effective communication strategies.

Communication Strategies

If your family does this:	Try to do this instead:
Call each other names.	Express anger without hurt.
Put each other down.	"I am angry that you did _____."
Interrupt each other.	Take turns; keep it short.
Criticize too much.	Point out the good and bad.

If your family does this:	Try to do this instead:
Get defensive.	Listen, then calmly disagree.
Lecture.	Tell it straight and short.
Look away from the speaker.	Make eye contact.
Slouch.	Sit up, look attentive.
Talk in sarcastic tone.	Talk in normal tone.
Get off the topic.	Finish one topic, then go on.
Think the worst.	Don't jump to conclusions.
Dredge up the past.	Stick to the present.
Read others' minds.	Ask others' opinions.
Command, order.	Request nicely.
Give the silent treatment.	Say what's bothering you.
Make light of something.	Take it seriously.
Deny you did it.	Admit you did it, or nicely explain you didn't.
Nag about small mistakes.	Admit no one is perfect; overlook small things.

From Robin, A.T. (1998). *ADHD in Adolescents: Diagnosis and Treatment.* Copyright 1998 by The Guilford Press. Reprinted with permission.

Don't underestimate the influence you can continue to have, even though the feedback you're getting from your child may suggest otherwise. How gratifying it was to me (this is Peg talking) when my oldest son, around age 25 in a public forum (a "roast" sponsored by my state school psychology association), acknowledged that he really did learn a lot about managing his attention problems from his mom and some of those strategies she taught him really did work! I would never have guessed it, judging by his demeanor at age 17.

Given that you're likely to retain some influence over your children at this stage, what can you do to ensure your suggestions will be heard and—more important—that this advice will continue to foster the development of executive skills and independence? Throughout this book, we've stressed the importance of the child's active involvement in the problem-solving process. This is especially critical in the transition to adulthood. If you're to be an effective teacher for your adolescent, you'll have to assume a role somewhere between parent and coach. The relationship is collaborative, and the adolescent is encouraged to look at alternatives and make choices and decisions. From a parent's point of view, this process of having the child gather information, generate options, and collaborate on decisions may not seem (or be) efficient. The goal is not an efficient, parent-generated, solution, even though this might satisfy the immediate need of the child and the parent. The goal is for the parent to provide a framework that the child, through repeated experiences, can use as his or her own.

Your child is more likely to hear what you have to say if you can talk about your own struggles in this transition to adulthood. This can give you the opportunity to discuss general problem areas such as budgeting and money management, being on time for work, going to class, handling difficult bosses/coworkers, and so forth. By now, you'll also be well aware of your child's executive skill weaknesses and the situations that are most troublesome. So you can also use the occasion to plant a seed about which situations are probably going to be difficult. The information is more likely to be heard if you present it in a casual way and then leave it for your child to ponder, rather than as a lecture or a lesson. The lesson will come from the real-life experience and not from your warning anyway. When the struggle or failure does come, you'll have to resist the "I told you so" urge. If you can do that, a problem-solving discussion is still possible.

Once children depart home and high school for their next step into the world (college, job, service), they face some immediate challenges including budgeting, planning, time and money management, and impulse control in the face of new opportunities. At the same time, they gain an advantage that up until now has been quite limited. That advantage is expanded choice. Throughout childhood and early adolescence, many choices are made for children, and school is their primary "job." If their executive skills are not a good match for the demands they face, there is little that they can do about it. However, once they finish high school and leave home, they have much greater control over what they choose to do.

When youngsters have some awareness of their strong and weak executive skills, they can begin to select themselves in or out of situations and tasks based on whether their skills are a good "fit" for the demands. You can assist this process by talking with your child about his strong and weak skills. You can also point out how your child's skills are likely to match up against certain demands. For example, the adolescent with organization or time management weaknesses or inattention to detail is apt to be challenged by the need to monitor a bank balance or to submit license or car registration renewals on time. If flexibility is a weakness, a job that requires changing schedules or varying responsibilities will cause problems. Depending on the choices or tasks taken on by the child, you will also have an idea of where your support will be most needed.

In the transition to adulthood, *experiences* in the real world have a far greater impact on behavior than speeches or admonitions from parents. However, being free to test reality can feel risky to your child and to you. As we noted earlier in this book, this is a generation of young adults who are close to their parents. The converse is also true: today's parents feel close to their children. For this reason, you may feel more reluctant to let reality teach the lessons. We work to prevent our children from experiencing unpleasant situations, rejection, and failure. This may be part of the reason that so many children are unprepared for the transition to adulthood, a point made persuasively by Mel Levine in his book *Ready or Not, Here Life Comes*. Instead of trying to prevent rejection or failure, we can, along with Henry Ford, see it as an opportunity: "Failure is only opportunity to more intelligently begin again."

Fortunately, you have strategies you can use with your adolescent and young adult children that will help them experience and learn from reality without feeling like you've simply thrown them off the dock. One strategy is to actively bring youngsters into any task or situation that ultimately they will have to manage on their own. Having them go to banks to investigate car loans, calculate their education expenses and debt, and develop a budget for an apartment, living expenses, and car payments are important learning experiences. They get the opportunity to match their own ideas against reality in a context where someone other than parents is providing the information.

One parent recently told us of his daughter's plan to start her own business. His attempts to point out her "unrealistic" expectations and warn her off only made her more determined. Seeing that his attempt to save her from herself would not work, he offered to help in whatever way he could. Together they identified the information she would need, and she was able to meet with a real estate agent about what a small shop would cost and then get prices about expenses and inventory. She hasn't yet decided if she wants to or can pursue her idea, but the experience has been valuable and her father feels more confident about her choices.

A second, and in the short run somewhat more painful, strategy is to let the child fail. This is not a new strategy for parents. Throughout development, you've let your child experience failure in order to help the child learn frustration tolerance and persistence in problem solving. The consequences can be a little greater once your child is away from home, but the objective remains the same. Getting a ticket for an unregistered vehicle or for speeding, paying charges for an overdrawn account, having a debit card rejected while waiting for food, and paying for a lost cell phone (iPod, car key, license) create a level of awareness that parents' words simply cannot match. While these and other experiences may not completely correct a problem, the impact of repeated consequences can be a powerful agent for behavior change.

To use this strategy effectively, you need to be sure that the failure experiences do not occur with such frequency or severity that the child becomes discouraged. To ensure this, you'll want to use a slight modification of an earlier teaching principle—provide the minimum support necessary for children to be successful. The new principle becomes: Provide the least support necessary for them to pick themselves up and dust themselves off after they have made a mistake so they can continue on their journey toward independence.

For all of us, but particularly for children with executive skill weaknesses, failures are inevitable. Because of this, a pure "tough love, sink or swim" approach can be risky. In our work, parents and children have been most successful when parents have combined teaching strategies with ongoing, gradually decreasing support as children show increasingly more success in handling adult responsibilities.

Parting Thoughts

If you read this book from cover to cover, your head may be reeling. That IM acronym, TMI, comes to mind—too much information! At least too much to absorb easily. We'll leave you with a quick review of what we see as the most important things you can do:

- Identify strengths and weaknesses in executive skills and the circumstances in which they occur. Discuss these with your children so they can begin to see and label them.
- Start working on strategies as early as possible, but remember that whenever you start, your children will benefit.
- Help children learn how to make an effort by using small steps, reinforcing their attempts and only gradually fading your coaching.
- Point them toward resources (people, experiences, books) that they can access for advice/help when they are ready.
- Decide what type of support you can give (money, time, living situation), for how long and under what conditions.
- Let children know, specifically, what their end of the bargain is (financial contribution, grades, work at home).
- If they fall behind in keeping an agreement, discuss this openly and in a timely fashion. The rest of the world (bosses, professors, etc.) will pay attention to their performance, and you should too.
- If they fail, offer an understanding word and help if they cannot get back on track. Remember that if they want to manage on their own, seek help only when they decide it is needed, and do not want to be rescued by you, this is a positive sign.
- As always, encourage their efforts, praise their successes, and let them know that you love them.

Resources

Books

Baker, B. L., & Brightman, A. J. (2004). *Steps to Independence: Teaching Everyday Skills to Children with Special Needs*. Baltimore: Brookes.—Written for parents of children aged 3 or older, this book provides an overview of teaching principles, followed by a step-by-step guide to teaching seven different types of skills: get-ready, self-help, toilet training, play, self-care, home-care, and information-gathering skills.

Barkley, R. A. (1997). *ADHD and the Nature of Self-Control*. New York: Guilford Press.—This book is fairly technical but provides a good description of executive skills within a developmental framework and argues that executive skills are at the core of ADHD. Russell Barkley has written a number of other books that parents may find helpful, especially parents of defiant children or those with ADHD. These include:

- *Taking Charge of ADHD (rev. ed.): The Complete Authoritative Guide for Parents*. New York: Guilford Press, 2000.
- *Your Defiant Child: Eight Steps to Better Behavior* (coauthored by Christine Benton). New York: Guilford Press, 1998.
- *Your Defiant Teen: 10 Steps to Resolve Conflict and Rebuild Your Relationship* (coauthored by Arthur Robin). New York: Guilford Press, 2008.

Buron, K. D., & Curtis, M. (2003). *The Incredible 5-Point Scale*. Shawnee Mission, KS: Autism Aspergers Publishing Company.—This brief book, written by a couple of special education teachers, describes how to use rating scales to help children learn to understand and control their emotions.

Dawson, P., & Guare, R. (1998). *Coaching the ADHD Student*. North Tonawanda, NY: Multi-Health Systems.—This manual describes in some detail the coaching process, an intervention strategy ideally designed to help teenagers build stronger executive skills.

Dawson, P., & Guare, R. (2004). *Executive Skills in Children and Adolescents: A Practical Guide to Assessment and Intervention*. New York: Guilford Press.—This book, written primarily for educators and school psychologists, describes how executive skills are assessed but also provides descriptions of school-based interventions for executive skill weaknesses following the same framework that we describe in this volume.

Ginott, H. (2003). *Between Parent and Child*. New York: Three Rivers Press.—This is an updated edition of a classic book. It's the best book we know of on how to communicate with children in ways that encourage confidence and competence.

Goldberg, D. (2005). *The Organized Student: Teaching Children the Skills for Success in School and Beyond*. New York: Fireside.—Lots of hands-on strategies from an educational consultant who developed them by working with students, including plans for keeping a backpack organized, managing school binders, arranging study space at home, and managing time.

Goldberg, E. (2001). *The Executive Brain: Frontal Lobes and the Civilized Mind*. New York: Oxford University Press.—A somewhat technical but very readable description of how the frontal lobes of the brain control judgment and decision making. For people who want a more thorough description of research delineating executive skills, this is an excellent resource.

Greene, R. W. (2001). *The Explosive Child: A New Approach for Understanding and Parenting Easily Frustrated, Chronically Inflexible Children*. New York: Harper Collins.—This very readable book is a source of comfort to parents of inflexible children, as it describes the causes of inflexibility as well as ways to treat the problem in clear, straightforward language.

Harvey, V. S. & Chickie-Wolfe, L. A. (2007). *Fostering Independent Learning: Practical Strategies to Promote Student Success*. New York: Guilford Press.—This book, written primarily for educators and school psychologists, describes strategies to help students become independent learners. There is considerable overlap with the concepts described in our book, and parents may be able to use some of the strategies described by Harvey and Chickie-Wolfe.

Huebner, D. (2006). *What to Do When You Worry Too Much: A Kid's Guide to Overcoming Anxiety*. Washington, DC: Magination Press.—This is one of a series of books written by a therapist that are designed to help children manage their emotions more successfully. Other books by the same author are:

- *What to Do When You Grumble Too Much: A Kid's Guide to Overcoming Negativity*. Washington, DC: Magination Press, 2006.
- *What to Do When Your Brain Gets Stuck: A Kid's Guide to Overcoming OCD*. Washington, DC: Magination Press, 2007.
- *What to Do When Your Temper Flares: A Kid's Guide to Overcoming Problems with Anger*. Washington, DC: Magination Press, 2008.

Kurcinka, M. S. (2006). *Raising Your Spirited Child*. New York: Harper.—The author describes spirited children as "intense, sensitive, perceptive, persistent, and energetic." The book helps parents understand the role of temperament in the behavior of their children and offers advice for how to handle common problems of daily living with children who have problems with emotional control and response inhibition.

Kutscher, M. L. (2005). *Kids in the Syndrome Mix of ADHD, LD, Asperger's, Tourette's, Bipolar and More!* London: Jessica Kingsley.—This book, written by a psychiatrist for parents, teachers, and other professionals, is a concise guide to a range of neurobehavioral disorders in children, most of which involve executive skill deficits. It includes tips for managing children at home and in the classroom and includes a chapter on commonly prescribed medications.

Landry, S. H., Miller-Loncar, C. L., Smith, K. E., & Swank, P. R. (2002). The role of early parenting in children's development of executive processes. *Developmental Neuropsychology, 21,* 15–41.

Levine, M. (2002). *A Mind at a Time.* New York: Simon & Schuster.—Mel Levine has written many books parents may find helpful. We like this one the best. Here, he describes eight different brain "systems," the roles they play in learning, and how parents and teachers can take advantage of learning strengths and bypass weaknesses to help children be successful students. A PBS documentary describes Dr. Levine's work (available at *www.pbs.org/wgbh/misunderstoodminds*).

Levine, M. (2005). *Ready or Not, Here Life Comes.* New York: Simon & Schuster.

Martin, C., Dawson, P., & Guare, R. (2007). *Smarts: Are We Hardwired for Success?* New York: AMACOM.—This book applies the same executive skills construct to an adult population, particularly focusing on workplace issues and how people can take advantage of their executive skill strengths and work around their weaknesses to function more effectively on the job.

Rief, S. F. (1997). *The ADD/ADHD Checklist.* San Francisco: Jossey-Bass.—This book contains descriptions of deep breathing, progressive relaxation, and other self-soothing techniques that you can teach your child.

Robin, A. T., (1998). *ADHD in Adolescents: Diagnosis and Treatment.* New York: Guilford Press.

Schaefer, C. E., & DiGeronimo, T. F. (2000). *Ages and Stages: A Parent's Guide to Normal Childhood Development.* New York: Wiley.—This book provides an excellent guide for parents about normal child development, and includes, according to the book's authors "tips and techniques for building your child's social, emotional, interpersonal, and cognitive skills.

Shure, M. B. (2001). *I Can Problem Solve: An Interpersonal Cognitive Problem-Solving Program: Preschool.* Champaign, IL: Research Press.

Magazines

ADDitude is a magazine for families affected by ADHD. Every issue includes articles on a range of topics, many of which relate to executive skills, including product reviews, practical advice, and helpful suggestions for managing ADHD in children and adults. They also offer a helpful website (*www.additudemag.com*).

Attention! is the official publication of CHADD (Children and Adults with Attention Deficit/Hyperactivity Disorder). It serves the same audience served by *ADDitude* and contains similar practical articles. They, too, have a useful website (*www.chadd.org*).

Parents magazine offers general advice on child development and parenting issues. Their website is *www.parents.com*.

Toys and Other Devices to Promote Executive Skill Development

Cueing and Time Management Devices

Time Timer (*www.timetimer.com*), available in a desktop or computer version, helps children understand time by providing a graphic depiction of time passing. Its use can help children learn to monitor work production and build time management skills.

WatchMinder (*www.watchminder.com*) is a programmable watch that can be set with daily alarms and preprogrammed messages. Can be used for self-monitoring and for cueing children to remember important events or tasks.

MotivAider is a device that periodically vibrates to remind children to ask themselves whether they are paying attention (or staying on task). Because it fits in a child's pocket and can't be heard by others, it protects the child's privacy while providing reminders. A more public (and more costly) device called the Attention Training System Starter Package sits on the child's desk and automatically awards the child a point every 60 seconds, with remote controls for teacher or parents to deduct points and turn on a warning light if the child gets off-task. This system is more suited for classroom use because the teacher can monitor up to four students at a time with it, but you may find it useful too. Available from the A.D.D. WareHouse (*www.addwarehouse.com*), which also sells numerous books, games, and other tools for use with kids who have problems related to ADHD.

Toys and Games

MindWare (*www.mindwareonline.com*), a catalogue of "brainy toys for kids of all ages," offers a wide variety of toys designed to build creativity and problem solving (that is, metacognitive skills).

Childswork/Childsplay (*www.childswork.com*) is a catalog of games and activities primarily designed for guidance counselors and therapists to help children learn to recognize and manage their feelings. Most of the materials are not restricted to professionals and may be helpful for parents who want to work on emotional control with their children.

SmileMakers (*www.smilemakers.com*) offers a wide array of low-cost reinforcers such as stickers and inexpensive toys that could be used for home reward systems.

Office Playground (*www.officeplayground.com*) is an online catalog of toys and gadgets (for example, stress balls, desktop toys, sand timers, etc.) that can be used as reinforcers or can be used to help children manage emotions such as anger and anxiety.

The Relaxation Station (*www.therelaxationstation.com*) is a 2-hour DVD that provides exercises and calming images to help children learn relaxation techniques. Developed by the Children's Hospital of Michigan for hospitalized kids, it has been shown in studies to help children (and their parents!) with a wide variety of needs soothe and calm themselves.

Websites

About Kids Health (*www.aboutkidshealth.ca*), developed by The Hospital for Sick Children in Toronto, is a valuable source of information on topics involving child health, behavior and development. The series on executive skills in children is excellent.

American Academy of Pediatrics (*www.aap.org*), the official website of the American Academy of Pediatrics, is an excellent source of information about all aspects of children's health. Check this site for information on relaxation techniques for children.

Autism Research Centre (*www.autismresearchcentre.com*), is an excellent source of information on research into autism spectrum disorders and the deficits in "theory of mind" and the related executive skills that children with these disorders typically experience.

Based at Cambridge University in England and directed by preeminent scholar and researcher Simon Baron-Cohen, PhD.

Autism Research Institute (ARI) (*www.autism.com*) has devoted its work to conducting research, and to disseminating the results of research, on the triggers of autism and on methods of diagnosing and treating autism. It provides research-based information to parents and professionals around the world. Search the site for recent articles related to executive skills/functions.

Autism Society of America (*www.autism-society.org*) is a national grassroots organization dedicated to promoting advocacy, education, support, services, and research for individuals on the autism spectrum including Asperger syndrome. It provides reliable, up-to-date information about autism spectrum disorders. A wealth of articles on educational approaches appropriate to addressing the executive skill weaknesses present in autism.

Autism Society Canada (*www.autismsocietycanada.ca*) is committed to advocacy, public education, information and referral, and provincial development support.

Autism Speaks (*www.autismspeaks.org*) is dedicated to funding global biomedical research into the causes, prevention, treatments, and cure for autism; to raising public awareness about autism and its effects on individuals, families, and society; and to bringing hope to all who deal with the hardships of this disorder. Search for executive functions and executive skills.

Autism Spectrum Australia (*www.aspect.org.au*) is a nonprofit organization that provides information, education, and other services through partnerships with people with autism spectrum disorders, their families, and communities. Participates in research and offers an information line and a paid-subscription, interactive web-based service called Autism Pro that allows parents to work with professionals in choosing objectives and activities and designing intervention programs for their children with autism.

Autism Today (*www.canadianautism.com*) is a free-membership organization that offers access to over 5,000 articles and other resources and a store for purchasing books and additional tools on autism spectrum disorders. The organization also plans workshops and conferences to disseminate information and practical advice about autism spectrum disorders.

Brain Connection (*www.brainconnection.com*) provides a variety of articles and resources for parents and professionals about brain development and new brain research, particularly how these relate to children's learning.

Canadian Paediatric Society (*www.cps.ca/english*) serves members of the Canadian Paediatric Society and other health care professionals with information they need to make informed decisions about child health care. Parents, journalists, and others involved in the care of children will also find the site useful.

CanChild Centre for Childhood Disability Research (*www.canchild.ca*) is a research and educational center. The majority of its research work is focused on issues that make a difference for children and youth with physical, developmental, and communication needs and their families.

Centers for Disease Control and Prevention (CDC) (*www.cdc.gov*), part of the U.S. Department of Health and Human Services, is the primary federal agency for conducting and supporting public health activities in the United States. The site contains links to research studies on executive skills/functions in children as well as comprehensive information on disorders associated with executive skill deficits, including autism and ADHD.

CHADD (*www.chadd.org*) is an organization dedicated to providing advocacy, education, and support for individuals with ADHD. The website is an excellent source of information for individuals, parents, and professionals about topics related to ADHD.

Children's Technology Review (*www.childrenssoftware.com*) provides professional reviews of interactive technology (software, videogames) to help guide parents and professionals in monitoring and choosing products that children are exposed to daily.

Council for Exceptional Children (*www.cec.sped.org*) is an international, professional organization whose mission is to improve educational outcomes for students with disabilities, individuals with exceptionalities, and/or the gifted.

Early Childhood Australia (*www.earlychildhood.org.au*) a broad-based, private nonprofit advocacy organization full of information and resources for parents and educators, addressing developmental needs of children up to age 8.

Exploring Autism (*www.exploringautism.org*) is the result of a collaboration between researchers, nonprofit groups, and families who are living with autism. Focusing on the genetics of autism, the site contains a lot of information about brain development.

Family Education (*www.familyeducation.com*) is a website that's packed with information, parenting tips, and family games and activities aimed at parents of children from birth to age 18.

Gray Center for Social Learning and Understanding (*www.thegraycenter.org*) is an organization devoted to promoting understanding between individuals on the autism spectrum and those who work alongside them. The site is an excellent source of information about the development of social stories that parents and professionals can use as teaching tools with all children.

Intervention Central (*www.interventioncentral.org*) offers a wide range of tools and resources for parents and school staffs to promote effective learning and positive classroom behavior for children.

LD OnLine (*www.ldonline.org*) provides up-to-date information and advice about learning disabilities and ADHD, serving more than 200,000 parents, teachers, and other professionals each month. The site features hundreds of helpful articles, multimedia, monthly columns by noted experts, first-person essays, children's writing and artwork, a comprehensive resource guide, very active forums, and a yellow pages referral directory of professionals, schools, and products.

Learning Disabilities Association of America (*www.ldanatl.org*) is an organization dedicated to promoting an understanding of learning disabilities, creating success for individuals with learning disabilities, and reducing the incidence of these disabilities in the future. This is a comprehensive site for information about all aspects of learning disabilities.

Learning Disabilities Association of Canada (*www.ldac-taac.ca*) is a private nonprofit organization whose members are mostly parents but also professionals whose mission is to serve as the Canadian national voice for individuals with learning disabilities and those who support them. The association publishes books and other materials containing a broad range of information, practical help, and news in the field, and the site contains numerous links to other organizations in Canada and worldwide, other publications, and legal assistance.

MAAP Services (*www.maapservices.org*) is dedicated to providing information and advice to families of more advanced (high-functioning) individuals with autism, Asperger syndrome, and pervasive developmental disorder (PDD).

MyADHD (*www.myadhd.com*) is a subscription website that offers tools for assessment, treatment, and progress monitoring, as well as a library of articles, audio programs, and charts that parents can use to better understand and manage their children's attention disorder.

My Reward Board (*www.myrewardboard.com*) is a website containing chore lists and reward charts in a variety of formats. Points can be earned for completing chores and deposited in "bank accounts" for later withdrawal. The program emphasizes a positive approach for encouraging kids to complete their chores, achieve their goals, improve their behavior, and save their money. A 15-day free trial is available prior to purchase.

National Autistic Society, United Kingdom (*www.nas.org.uk*) is a nonprofit parents' organization dedicated to providing a wide range of services and information for U.K. families with children diagnosed with an autism spectrum disorder, from schools and outreach services to social and respite support, research data, diagnostic and treatment information, and parent courses and training. Based in London, the society has chapters throughout the United Kingdom.

National Center for Learning Disabilities (*www.ncld.org*) is a parent-led organization that promotes research and programs to facilitate effective learning, advocates for educational rights and opportunities, and provides information to parents, professionals, and individuals with learning disabilities.

National Institute of Child Health and Human Development (NICHD) (*www.nichd.nih. gov*) supports and conducts research and clinical work on the neurobiological, developmental, and behavioral processes that affect children and families. Provides authoritative information about a broad range of child health and behavioral issues.

PBS (*www.pbs.org*) has provided and continues to provide excellent, scientifically based programming on child health and development including brain-behavior relationships.

PTA (*www.pta.org*) provides parents with extensive information and resources about topics such as student achievement, safety, media technology and nutrition, and health and wellness.

Psychiatric Times (*www.psychiatrictimes.com*) is an authoritative, monthly online publication offering feature articles and clinical news and reports on special topics across a broad range of psychiatric issues involving children and adults.

Smart Kids with Learning Disabilities (*www.smartkidswithld.org*) is a valuable source of information, support, and encouragement for parents of children with learning disabilities and attention deficit disorders.

Specific Learning Disabilities Federation (SPELD) New Zealand (*www.speld.org.nz*) is a nonprofit advocacy organization dedicated to those with learning disabilities, including LDs associated with attention disorders and autism spectrum disorders, via chapters throughout New Zealand. The federation's main objectives are in advocacy, assessment and tutoring, and family support. Offers courses and certification to train teachers and parents as learning disabilities tutors.

Thanet ADDers (*www.adders.org/thanet.htm*) is a support-group resource based in Kent, England, and operated by a parent of an adult diagnosed with ADD who also has the disorder herself. She offers links for buying books and other resources, support and information, and provides "as much free practical help" as possible to those dealing with ADD and ADHD.

Wrightslaw (*www.wrightslaw.com*) contains articles focusing on special education law and advocacy for children with disabilities.

Zero to Three (*www.zerotothree.org*) provides authoritative information on a host of topics (brain development, nutrition, child rearing) for adults who influence the lives of infants and toddlers.

Index

About the Authors

Peg Dawson, EdD, is a staff psychologist at the Center for Learning and Attention Disorders, in Portsmouth, New Hampshire. Dr. Dawson is a past president of both the National Association of School Psychologists and the International School Psychology Association. She is a recipient of the National Association of School Psychologists' Lifetime Achievement Award.

Richard Guare, PhD, is a neuropsychologist and Director of the Center for Learning and Attention Disorders. His research and publications focus on understanding and treatment of learning and attention difficulties and neurological disorders. Board certified as a behavior analyst, Dr. Guare frequently consults to schools and agencies.

Drs. Dawson and Guare have over 30 years of experience working with children with learning, attention, and behavior difficulties. Together, they are the authors of *Executive Skills in Children and Adolescents*, a practical guide for school professionals.